Marcia Finlayson, PhD, OT(C), OTR/L
Editor

Occupational Therapy Practice and Research with Persons with Multiple Sclerosis

Occupational Therapy Practice and Research with Persons with Multiple Sclerosis has been co-published simultaneously as *Occupational Therapy in Health Care*, Volume 17, Numbers 3/4 2003.

Pre-publication
REVIEWS,
COMMENTARIES,
EVALUATIONS . . .

"AN IMPORTANT RESOURCE FOR STUDENTS, CLINICIANS, AND RESEARCHERS who work with and/or study persons with MS. This collection will help us understand the unique needs of persons, especially the aging, with MS. A moving testimonial by a consumer of OT services helps us understand the important role that OT can play in improving the quality of life of persons with MS when we use a client-centered, occupation-based approach to treatment."

Virgil Mathiowetz, PhD, OTR/L, FAOTA
Associate Professor
Program in Occupational Therapy
University of Minnesota, Minneapolis

Occupational Therapy Practice and Research with Persons with Multiple Sclerosis

Occupational Therapy Practice and Research with Persons with Multiple Sclerosis has been co-published simultaneously as *Occupational Therapy in Health Care*, Volume 17, Numbers 3/4 2003.

Occupational Therapy in Health Care Monographic "Separates"

Below is a list of "separates," which in serials librarianship means a special issue simultaneously published as a special journal issue or double-issue _and_ as a "separate" hardbound monograph. (This is a format which we also call a "DocuSerial.")

"Separates" are published because specialized libraries or professionals may wish to purchase a specific thematic issue by itself in a format which can be separately cataloged and shelved, as opposed to purchasing the journal on an on-going basis. Faculty members may also more easily consider a "separate" for classroom adoption.

"Separates" are carefully classified separately with the major book jobbers so that the journal tie-in can be noted on new book order slips to avoid duplicate purchasing.

You may wish to visit Haworth's website at . . .

http://www.HaworthPress.com

. . . to search our online catalog for complete tables of contents of these separates and related publications.

You may also call 1-800-HAWORTH (outside US/Canada: 607-722-5857), or Fax: 1-800-895-0582 (outside US/Canada: 607-771-0012), or e-mail at:

docdelivery@haworthpress.com

Occupational Therapy Practice and Research with Persons with Multiple Sclerosis, edited by Marcia Finlayson, PhD, OT(C), OTR/L (Vol. 17, No. 3/4, 2003). _Explores the complex OT issues arising from multiple sclerosis and suggests ways to enhance OT practice or research with people with MS._

Interprofessional Collaboration in Occupational Therapy, edited by Stanley Paul, PhD, and Cindee Q. Peterson, PhD, OTR (Vol. 15, No. 3/4, 2001). _"A GOOD SOURCE OF INFORMATION. . . . Introduces the reader to the concept of interprofessional collaboration, its benefits, barriers, and strategies for developing such collaboration. . . . Presents a series of research studies that show the value of interprofessional collaboration to achieve outcomes at different levels and within different service delivery models."_ (Dyhalma Irizarry, PhD, OTR/L, FAOTA, Director, Occupational Therapy Program, University of Puerto Rico)

Education for Occupational Therapy in Health Care: Strategies for the New Millennium, edited by Patricia Grist, PhD, OTR/L, FAOTA, and Marjorie Scaffa, PhD, OTR/L, FAOTA (Vol. 15, No. 1/2, 2001). _"PROVIDES TRULY IMAGINATIVE IDEAS for preparing the practitioners of the near future–and not a moment too soon! It is easy to see that these authors have been outstanding clinicians. . . . they put their OT skills to work in creating these unique learning-by-doing educational packages. Especially exciting are the clever ways in which alternative sites and programs are used to provide fieldwork experiences."_ (Nedra P. Gillette, MEd, OTR, ScD (Hon), Director, Institute for the Study of Occupation and Health, American Occupational Therapy Foundation)

Community Occupational Therapy Education and Practice, edited by Beth P. Velde, PhD, OTR/L, and Peggy Prince Wittman, EdD, OTR/L, FAOTA (Vol. 13, No. 3/4, 2001). _"Introduces the concept of community-based practice in non-traditional settings. Whether one is concerned with wellness and the aging process or with debilitating situations, injuries, or diseases such as homelessness, AIDS, or multiple sclerosis, this collection details the process of moving forward."_ (Scott D. McPhee, DrPH, OT, FAOTA, Associate Dean and Chair, School of Occupational Therapy, Belmont University, Nashville, Tennessee)

Occupational Therapy Practice and Research with Persons with Multiple Sclerosis

Marcia Finlayson, PhD, OT(C), OTR/L
Editor

Occupational Therapy Practice and Research with Persons with Multiple Sclerosis has been co-published simultaneously as *Occupational Therapy in Health Care*, Volume 17, Numbers 3/4 2003.

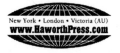

The Haworth Press, Inc.

New York • London • Victoria (AU)
www.HaworthPress.com

BS

Occupational Therapy Practice and Research with Persons with Multiple Sclerosis has been co-published simultaneously as *Occupational Therapy in Health Care™*, Volume 17, Numbers 3/4 2003.

Cover design by Brooke Stiles

Library of Congress Cataloging-in-Publication Data

Occupational therapy practice and research with persons with multiple sclerosis / Marcia Finlayson, editor.
    p. ; cm.
Simultaneously published as Occupational therapy in health care v. 17, no. 3/4 2003.
Includes bibliographical references and index.
ISBN 0-7890-2380-6 (hard cover : alk. paper) – ISBN 0-7890-2381-4 (soft cover : alk. paper)
    1. Multiple sclerosis–Patients–Rehabilitation. 2. Occupational therapy. I. Finlayson, Marcia.
[DNLM: 1. Multiple Sclerosis–rehabilitation. 2. Occupational Therapy–methods. WL 360 O15 2003]
RC377.O24 2003
616.8'3406515–dc22

                                              2003019802

9/8/04

Indexing, Abstracting & Website/Internet Coverage

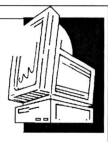

This section provides you with a list of major indexing & abstracting services. That is to say, each service began covering this periodical during the year noted in the right column. Most Websites which are listed below have indicated that they will either post, disseminate, compile, archive, cite or alert their own Website users with research-based content from this work. (This list is as current as the copyright date of this publication.)

Abstracting, Website/Indexing Coverage . . . . Year When Coverage Began

* *Abstracts in Social Gerontology: Current Literature on Aging* **1989**

* *Academic Abstracts/CD-ROM* **1995**

* *Biology Digest (in print & online)* **1990**

* *Biosciences Information Service of Biological Abstracts (BIOSIS),*
  a centralized source of life science information
  <http://www.biosis.org> . . . . *

* *Brandon/Hill Selected List of Journals in Allied Health Sciences* . . . **2000**

* *Cambridge Scientific Abstracts (Health & Safety Science Abstracts)*
  <http://www.csa.com> **1985**

* *CINAHL (Cumulative Index to Nursing & Allied Health*
  Literature) <http://www.cinahl.com> **1987**

* *CNPIEC Reference Guide: Chinese National Directory*
  of Foreign Periodicals **1995**

* *EMBASE/Excerpta Medica Secondary Publishing Division*
  <http://www.elsevier.nl>. **1985**

(continued)

- *Environmental Sciences and Pollution Management (Cambridge Scientific Abstracts Internet Database Service) <http://www.csa.com>* .... *

- *ERIC Clearinghouse on Disabilities & Gifted Education* 1985

- *Exceptional Child Education Resources (ECER), (CD/ROM from SilverPlatter and hard copy)* 1985

- *Health Source: Indexing & Abstracting of 160 selected health related journals, updated monthly: EBSCO Publishing* 1995

- *Health Source Plus: Expanded version of "Health Source": EBSCO Publishing* 1995

- *Human Resources Abstracts (HRA)* 1989

- *Index Guide to College Journals (core list compiled by integrating 48 indexes frequently used to support undergraduate programs in small to medium-sized libraries)* 1999

- *MANTIS (Manual, Alternative & Natural Therapy) <http://www.healthindex.com>* 1999

- *Occupational Therapy Database (OTDBASE) <http://www.otdbase.com>* 1993

- *Occupational Therapy Index/AMED Database* 1993

- *OCLC ArticleFirst <http://www.oclc.org/services/databases/>* .... *

- *OCLC ContentsFirst <http://www.oclc.org/services/databases/>* .... *

- *OT SEARCH* 1991

- *OT seeker <http://www.otseeker.com>* 2002

- *Physiotherapy Evidence Database (PEDro) .... internet-based database of: a) articles describing evidence-based clinical trials in physiotherapy; b) systematic reviews of each; c) single-case experimental studies of efficacy of therapeutic interventions. <http://ptwww.cchs.usyd.edu.au/pedro>* 2001

- *Social Work Abstracts <http://www.silverplatter.com/catalog/swab.htm>* 1990

(continued)

- *SocIndex (EBSCO)* 2003

- *SPORTDiscus <http://www.sportquest.com>* 1991

- *SwetsNet <http://www.swetsnet.com>* 2001

- *Violence and Abuse Abstracts: A Review of Current Literature on Interpersonal Violence (VAA)* 1995

  * **Exact start date to come.**

Special Bibliographic Notes related to special journal issues (separates) and indexing/abstracting:

- indexing/abstracting services in this list will also cover material in any "separate" that is co-published simultaneously with Haworth's special thematic journal issue or DocuSerial. Indexing/abstracting usually covers material at the article/chapter level.
- monographic co-editions are intended for either non-subscribers or libraries which intend to purchase a second copy for their circulating collections.
- monographic co-editions are reported to all jobbers/wholesalers/approval plans. The source journal is listed as the "series" to assist the prevention of duplicate purchasing in the same manner utilized for books-in-series.
- to facilitate user/access services all indexing/abstracting services are encouraged to utilize the co-indexing entry note indicated at the bottom of the first page of each article/chapter/contribution.
- this is intended to assist a library user of any reference tool (whether print, electronic, online, or CD-ROM) to locate the monographic version if the library has purchased this version but not a subscription to the source journal.
- individual articles/chapters in any Haworth publication are also available through the Haworth Document Delivery Service (HDDS).

Occupational Therapy Practice and Research with Persons with Multiple Sclerosis

CONTENTS

Foreword: A Note of Appreciation
from a Grateful Recipient   xiii
  Carol A. Gaetjens, PhD

Preface: Perspectives of an MS Researcher   xv
  Nicholas G. LaRocca, PhD

Introduction: Occupational Therapy Practice and Research
with Persons with Multiple Sclerosis   1
  Marcia Finlayson, PhD, OT (C), OTR/L

Multiple Perspectives on the Health Service Need,
Use, and Variability Among Older Adults
with Multiple Sclerosis   5
  Marcia Finlayson, PhD, OT(C), OTR/L
  Toni Van Denend, BS
  Eynat Shevil, BSc

Analysis of Symptoms, Functional Impairments,
and Participation in Occupational Therapy
for Individuals with Multiple Sclerosis   27
  Letha J. Mosley, MEd, OTR/L
  Gregory P. Lee, PhD
  Mary L. Hughes, MD
  Charlotte Chatto, PT, MS

Self-Report Assessment of Fatigue in Multiple Sclerosis:
A Critical Evaluation   45
  Daphne Kos, MSc
  Eric Kerckhofs, PhD
  Pierre Ketelaer, MD
  Marijke Duportail, OT
  Guy Nagels, MD
  Marie D'Hooghe, MD
  Godelieve Nuyens, PhD

The Effect of Wheelchair Use on the Quality of Life
   of Persons with Multiple Sclerosis   63
      Rachel Devitt, BHSc, OT Reg (Ont)
      Betty Chau, BSc, OT Reg (Ont)
      Jeffrey W. Jutai, PhD, CPsych

Interference of Upper Limb Tremor on Daily Life Activities
   in People with Multiple Sclerosis   81
      Peter Feys, PT, PhD student
      Anders Romberg, PT
      Juhnai Ruutiainen, MD
      Pierre Ketelaer, MD

Developing and Implementing Lifestyle Management
   Programs© with People with Multiple Sclerosis   97
      Christa Roessler, AccOT BAppSc(OT)Cumb
      Jenny Barling, AccOT BAppSc(OT)Cumb
      Megan Dephoff, AccOT BHlthSc(OT)
      Terri Johnson, OTR BSc(OT)
      Susan Sweeney, BAppSc(OT)Cumb

In Their Own Words: Coping Processes Among Women
   Aging with Multiple Sclerosis   115
      Julie DalMonte, MS, OTR/L
      Marcia Finlayson, PhD, OT(C), OTR/L
      Christine Helfrich, PhD, OTR/L, FAOTA

Occupational Therapy Practice and Research with Persons
   with MS: Final Reflections   139
      Laura McKeown, BSc (Hons) OT, SROT (UK)
      Marcia Finlayson, PhD, OT (C), OTR/L

Index   143

ABOUT THE EDITOR

Marcia Finlayson, PhD, OT(C), OTR/L, is Assistant Professor in the Department of Occupational Therapy at the University of Illinois at Chicago. She received her baccalaureate degree in Medical Rehabilitation (Occupational Therapy) in 1987 from the University of Manitoba, and then worked in a varity of hospital and community settings primarily serving with older adults. She returned to the University of Manitoba to complete an MSc and a PhD in the Department of Community Health Sciences, finishing her studies in 1999.

Dr. Finlayson's research and scholarship focus on the patterns and predictors of the need for and use of health-related services among people who are aging with disability, particularly individuals with multiple sclerosis (MS). Together wth her colleagues and collaborators, Dr. Finlayson has received financial support for her work from the National Multiple Sclerosis Society, the National Institute of Disability and Rehabilitation Research, and the Canadian Institutes of Health Research. She has over 20 peer-reviewed publications in journals such as *Canadian Journal of Occupational Therapy, American Journal of Occupational Therapy, Canadian Journal on Aging, The Gerontologist, British Journal of Occupational Therapy, Journal of Health Services Research and Policy,* and the *Journal of Disability Policy Studies.* Her articles address issues related to the development, implementation and evaluation of a wide range of services for older adults and persons with MS.

In addition to her scholarly work, Dr. Finlayson has a long history of commitment to community and professional service activities. She served on the Board of Directors of the Multiple Sclerosis Society of Canada (Manitoba Division) from 1992 to 1998, acting as Chair for the Social Action Committee during the majority of this time. Her contributions to this organization were recognized through a Manitoba Division Award of Merit (1996) and a National Certificate of Merit (1999). In more recent years, Dr. Finlayson has been actively involved in the Greater Illinois Chapter of the National Multiple Sclerosis Society. She also serves as a member of the Seniors' Service Committee for Oak

Park Township. On a professional level, Dr. Finlayson serves on the review boards of both the Canadian and American journals of occupational therapy, and has provided grant reviews for the Canadian Occupational Therapy Foundation, the Langeloth Foundation, the Retirement Research Foundation, and the field-initiated grants program of the National Institute of Disability and Rehabilitation Research.

Foreword:
A Note of Appreciation
from a Grateful Recipient

Family history has it that I was born feisty, stubborn, and independent, and the first sentences I spoke were "me do it" and "by myself." These qualities stood me in good stead for many years. When I graduated from college, my father gave me my very own tool kit so I was prepared to fix anything, or so I thought.

But life changed dramatically in my twenties when I received a diagnosis of multiple sclerosis. Clearly there were new challenges that couldn't be fixed with my personal toolbox. On an existential and psychological level a major modification of my self-image was needed. I had to learn to ask for and receive help *graciously,* to be appropriately *dependent.* For help with these issues I sought the counsel of a professional social worker.

Now, in my fifties, after years of medical professionals who focused on parts of my disease, parts of my body, it has been a pleasure to discover the skills of occupational therapists. They saw my disease in the total context of my life. They helped me solve practical challenges while teaching me how to live safely, efficiently and independently. They taught me how to arrange my clothes, to use reachers and sock adapters, to dress sitting down to save energy, to move safely in the bathroom. Because of occupational therapists, I learned how to use a cane correctly, stand up from a chair, drive my van with hand controls, use a rolling walker,

Carol A. Gaetjens is Adjunct Faculty, School of Education and Social Policy, Northwestern University, Walter Annenberg Hall, 2120 Campus Drive, Evanston, IL 60208 (E-mail: cgaetjens1@comcast.net).

[Haworth co-indexing entry note]: "Foreword: A Note of Appreciation from a Grateful Recipient." Gaetjens, Carol A. Co-published simultaneously in *Occupational Therapy in Health Care* (The Haworth Press, Inc) Vol. 17, No. 3/4, 2003, pp. xvii-xviii; and: *Occupational Therapy Practice and Research with Persons with Multiple Sclerosis* (ed: Marcia Finlayson) The Haworth Press, Inc., 2003, pp. xiii-xiv. Single or multiple copies of this article are available for a fee from The Haworth Document Delivery Service [1-800-HAWORTH, 9:00 a.m. - 5:00 p.m. (EST). E-mail address: docdelivery@haworthpress.com].

a scooter and a wheelchair. I can prepare meals on my own because everything in my kitchen is arranged to save energy and ensure my safety. The list could go on and on.

This special volume dedicated to multiple sclerosis is exciting for several reasons. First, the course of MS for each individual is so different and unpredictable that only allied health professionals devoted to evaluating and helping people in the total context of their individual lives can be truly responsive. Second, often well meaning people look at people with MS and comment "but you look so well." The same people have trouble understanding MS fatigue. Anything that this groundbreaking issue can do to heighten understanding of the challenges of living with MS is welcomed.

Finally, thanks to all of you occupational therapists for significantly improving the quality of my everyday life and the lives of thousands like me who live with the challenge of multiple sclerosis.

Carol A. Gaetjens, PhD

Preface:
Perspectives of an MS Researcher

The MS field has evolved dramatically since the January morning in 1979 when I saw my first patient with MS. At that time there were no MS disease-modifying drugs, rehabilitation professionals worked with persons with MS reluctantly due to the progressive nature of their condition, and MS cognitive problems were generally swept under the rug. As the Director of our MS center, Labe Scheinberg, MD, put it, it was the age of "diagnose and adios," and most people were told to "go home and learn to live with it."

Today, we have five FDA-approved disease-modifying drugs with 150 clinical trials underway, MS is an important population for rehabilitation professionals, cognition has come out from under the rug, and MS care is much more proactive. Recent progress in research focused on genetic-based susceptibility to MS, the immune processes underlying the pathogenesis of MS and possibilities for neural repair suggests that we are on the brink of exciting new discoveries in MS. While the treatment of and future prospects for MS have never been better, once people leave the doctor's office, they are still faced with the challenge of "learning to live with it."

Occupational therapy has a pivotal role in helping persons with MS acquire the skills they need to maximize their potential and minimize the effects of MS. However, with some notable exceptions, occupational therapists have been absent from the arenas of MS research and publishing. The relative dearth of MS research and publications by occupational

---

Nicholas G. LaRocca is Director, Health Care Delivery and Policy Research, National Multiple Sclerosis Society, 733 Third Avenue, New York, NY 10017 (E-mail: nicholas.larocca@nmss.org).

[Haworth co-indexing entry note]: "Preface: Perspectives of an MS Researcher." LaRocca, Nicholas, G. Co-published simultaneously in *Occupational Therapy in Health Care* (The Haworth Press, Inc.) Vol. 17, No. 3/4, 2003, pp. xix-xx; and: *Occupational Therapy Practice and Research with Persons with Multiple Sclerosis* (ed: Marcia Finlayson) The Haworth Press, Inc., 2003, pp. xv-xvi. Single or multiple copies of this article are available for a fee from The Haworth Document Delivery Service [1-800-HAWORTH, 9:00 a.m. - 5:00 p.m. (EST). E-mail address: docdelivery@haworthpress.com].

xv

therapists has slowed progress in this area and left occupational therapy with a limited scientific foundation vis-à-vis MS.

Occupational therapists need to expand their research activities and disseminate to other professionals the nature of their work with persons with MS. This special volume helps to fill some of these gaps and suggests some future directions for the field:

- Increasing the dissemination of information to professionals outside occupational therapy,
- Working with multi-disciplinary research teams to help evaluate the real-life impact of MS treatments, and
- Implementing and publishing research focused on the work done by occupational therapists.

Occupational therapy can have a great impact on the lives of persons with MS, it is high time to better integrate that impact into the world of MS research and clinical practice.

Nicholas G. LaRocca, PhD

Introduction:
Occupational Therapy Practice
and Research with Persons
with Multiple Sclerosis

Marcia Finlayson, PhD, OT (C), OTR/L

Recent searches combining the terms "occupational therapy" and "multiple sclerosis" in the databases MEDLINE (1966-2003), CINAHL (1982-2003), and OTDBASE (1970-2003) revealed 44 unique articles published across 22 different peer-reviewed journals. The topics of these articles were wide-ranging and included (but were not exclusive to) fatigue management, assistive technology use, pain management, employment issues, health promotion, and the development and use of specific assessment tools. The breadth of topics addressed in these articles corresponds to descriptions about the role of occupational therapists when working with persons with multiple sclerosis (MS) presented on the National Multiple Sclerosis Society website (*www.nmss.org*) and in leading occupational therapy textbooks (Crepeau, Cohn & Boyt Schell, 2003; Pedretti & Early, 2001; Trombly & Radomski, 2002).

In reviewing the findings of these searches, two issues struck me. First, 44 articles over approximately 30 years represents about 1.5 arti-

Marcia Finlayson is Assistant Professor, Department of Occupational Therapy, University of Illinois at Chicago, 1919 W. Taylor Street, Chicago, IL 60612-7250 (E-mail: marciaf@uic.edu).

[Haworth co-indexing entry note]: "Introduction: Occupational Therapy Practice and Research with Persons with Multiple Sclerosis." Finlayson, Marcia. Co-published simultaneously in *Occupational Therapy in Health Care* (The Haworth Press, Inc.) Vol. 17, No. 3/4, 2003, pp. 1-4; and: *Occupational Therapy Practice and Research with Persons with Multiple Sclerosis* (ed: Marcia Finlayson) The Haworth Press, Inc., 2003, pp. 1-4. Single or multiple copies of this article are available for a fee from The Haworth Document Delivery Service [1-800-HAWORTH, 9:00 a.m. - 5:00 p.m. (EST). E-mail address: docdelivery@haworthpress.com].

http://www.haworthpress.com/store/product.asp?sku=J003
10.1300/J003v17n03_01

cles per year. This number seems exceedingly low given that persons with MS represent one of the largest groups of chronically ill clients seen by occupational therapists in both institutional and non-institutional settings (Rijken & Dekker, 1998). Second, 44 articles across 22 different journals has both positive and negative aspects. On the positive side, occupational therapists and their co-authors are reaching a broad audience. In fact, 14 of these 22 journals are not primarily targeted to occupational therapists. On the negative side, occupational therapists searching for information and evidence to support and develop their work with persons with multiple sclerosis will have a difficult time pulling together the relevant articles in the field, especially if they do not have access to a university library. Accessing information from other countries might be particularly difficult. These challenges are noteworthy in a climate where evidence-based practice is a critical factor in selecting individual interventions, determining funding allotments, setting strategic program directions, and making other programmatic and service decisions (Law, 2002; Taylor, 2000).

This special volume represents a small effort to address both of the low numbers of articles on occupational therapy and multiple sclerosis, and the challenges of finding a series of papers in one place. This volume includes seven international peer-reviewed papers about occupational therapy practice and research with persons with MS. The papers presented here come from Europe, Australia, Canada and the United States. I intentionally pursued international representation for this volume after attending meetings of the Consortium of Multiple Sclerosis Centers and the World Federation of Occupational Therapists in 2002. During these two events, I had the opportunity to meet and talk with occupational therapists from many countries who focus their clinical practices and/or research on the issues facing persons with MS. These discussions highlighted for me the incredible need to share international perspectives on MS and occupational therapy.

In addition to international representation, this volume also offers a second exciting feature that I did not intentionally pursue: Authors from disciplines beyond occupational therapy. As I was receiving submissions for this volume, I became aware that the authors and co-authors of the papers came not only from occupational therapy, but also from medicine, physical therapy and psychology. I see this diversity as a demonstration of the collaborative nature of service provision for persons with MS, and illustration that occupational therapists are valued members of MS research and care teams.

Across the articles in this volume, readers will learn about:

1. the perceived health-related service needs of older adults with MS,
2. the differences in the symptoms and functional limitations experienced by persons with MS who are referred occupational therapy compared to those who are not,
3. the range of fatigue assessment tools that are available for clinical and research applications,
4. the effect of wheelchair use on quality of life,
5. the implications of tremor on the everyday activities,
6. the development and use of Lifestyle Management Programs, and
7. coping processes used by women who are aging with MS.

Readers will find some repetition across the papers in terms of the descriptions of MS, and the symptoms and functional limitations experienced by persons with this disease. I chose to leave much (but not all) of this duplication since many of the articles will be read and used as individual, freestanding works. Consequently, I have chosen not to use this introduction to describe MS, its epidemiology, etiology, progression and treatments. Instead, the authors have included the basic information about MS that they needed to contextualize their own work.

While this volume does not and could not represent the diversity of topics that could be covered in such an issue, it does capture the complexity of issues arising from the MS disease process and suggests ways that occupational therapists can work with persons with MS to minimize their disabilities, enhance their quality of life, and promote their social and community participation. Across these articles physical and psychosocial issues are addressed, a range of methodological approaches are applied, and both narrative and numerical data are presented and interpreted. In addition, readers will find that both individual and system level issues emerge for occupational therapists to consider. Assessment and intervention ideas are offered, and information that could be used for broader program planning is also provided. I hope that all readers will be able to take something from this volume to enhance their practice or research with persons with MS.

In conclusion, this volume is the compilation of the work and contributions of many people. Special thanks go to the following people: Anne Dickerson for providing me with the opportunity to put together this collection and for answering my questions along the way; colleagues who graciously agreed to review the submissions for this volume, even though their schedules were already full; Alisa Bell, for her keen eye and orientation to details during the final editing of the papers; and all of the contributors without whom this volume could not have happened. I hope that through the information shared in these articles occupational therapy services for this population will be enhanced. I also hope that this collection will inspire others to write about their work with persons with MS so that next time I do a general search on "occupational therapy" and "multiple sclerosis" I will find much more than 44 unique articles.

REFERENCES

Crepeau, E.B., Cohn, E.S., & Boyt Schell, B.A. (2003). *Willard & Spackman's Occupational Therapy, 10th edition.* Philadelphia, PA: Lippincott Williams & Wilkins.

Law, M. (2002). *Evidence-based rehabilitation: A guide to practice.* Thorofare, NJ: Slack.

Pedretti, L.W., & Early, M.B. (2001). *Occupational therapy: Practice skills for physical dysfunction, 5th edition.* St. Louis, MO: Mosby.

Rijken, P.M., & Dekker, J. (1998). Clinical experience of rehabilitation therapists with chronic diseases: A quantitative approach. *Clinical Rehabilitation, 12,* 143-150.

Taylor, M.C. (2000). *Evidence-based practice for occupational therapists.* Osney Mead, Oxford: Blackwell Science.

Trombly, C.A., & Radomski, M.V. (2002). *Occupational therapy for physical dysfunction, 5th edition.* Philadelphia, PA: Lippincott Williams & Wilkins.

Multiple Perspectives
on the Health Service Need, Use,
and Variability Among Older Adults
with Multiple Sclerosis

Marcia Finlayson, PhD, OT(C), OTR/L
Toni Van Denend, MS
Eynat Shevil, BSc

SUMMARY. The purpose of this paper is to present the findings from the first phase of a large study that is examining the unmet health-related service needs of people aging with MS. Fifty-one volunteers participated

Marcia Finlayson is Assistant Professor, Department of Occupational Therapy, University of Illinois at Chicago, 1919 W. Taylor Street (MC 811), Chicago, IL 60612 (E-mail: marciaf@uic.edu). Toni Van Denend is Research Project Coordinator, Department of Occupational Therapy, University of Illinois at Chicago, 1919 W. Taylor Street (MC 811), Chicago, IL 60612 (E-mail: tvande2@uic.edu). Eynat Shevil is Research Assistant, Department of Occupational Therapy, University of Illinois at Chicago, 1919 W. Taylor Street (MC 811), Chicago, IL 60612 (E-mail: eshevil@uic.edu).

The authors would like to thank the members of the Study Advisory Group and the staff at the National Multiple Sclerosis Society Chapters in Minnesota, Wisconsin, Illinois, Indiana and Michigan for their assistance with recruiting participants for focus groups.

This study is supported by the National Multiple Sclerosis Society through Health Care Delivery and Policy Research Contract #HC049, awarded to Dr. Finlayson.

The information presented in this paper does not necessarily reflect the position, ideas or opinions of the National Multiple Sclerosis Society.

[Haworth co-indexing entry note]: "Multiple Perspectives on the Health Service Need, Use, and Variability Among Older Adults with Multiple Sclerosis." Finlayson, Marcia, Toni Van Denend, and Eynat Shevil. Co-published simultaneously in *Occupational Therapy in Health Care* (The Haworth Press, Inc.) Vol. 17, No. 3/4, 2003, pp. 5-25; and: *Occupational Therapy Practice and Research with Persons with Multiple Sclerosis* (ed: Marcia Finlayson) The Haworth Press, Inc., 2003, pp. 5-25. Single or multiple copies of this article are available for a fee from The Haworth Document Delivery Service [1-800-HAWORTH, 9:00 a.m. - 5:00 p.m. (EST). E-mail address: docdelivery@haworthpress.com].

in seven focus groups–five with individuals with MS and their family members, and two with health care professionals. Content analysis indicated health promotion (both physical and social), community accessibility, and support to remain at home as the most commonly identified health-related service needs. Differences were observed between the groups of individuals with MS/family members and health professionals. Findings point to the importance of using a client-centered approach when working with persons with multiple sclerosis and their family members. *[Article copies available for a fee from The Haworth Document Delivery Service: 1-800-HAWORTH. E-mail address: <docdelivery@haworthpress.com> Website: <http://www.HaworthPress.com> © 2003 by The Haworth Press, Inc. All rights reserved.]*

KEYWORDS. Health-related service needs, multiple sclerosis, focus groups, older adults

INTRODUCTION

Multiple Sclerosis (MS) is a chronic, debilitating neurological disease. Although MS can result in considerable disability, it does not significantly reduce life expectancy unless the impairments associated with the disease are severe (Miller, Hornabrook, & Purdie, 1992; Weinshenker, 1995). Eighty-five to ninety percent of individuals who are diagnosed with MS in their early 20s are likely to live for 50 or more years (Weinshenker, 1995), based on current life expectancy estimates in the United States. Consequently, these individuals will be required to manage MS-related disability at the same time they are dealing with changes related to normal aging. Although the interaction between aging and MS is unknown, it is likely to have important implications for how older persons with MS function, and for the types of services they need over time. Despite this, few researchers have examined the health-related service needs of older adults with MS. The purpose of this paper is to present the findings from the first phase of a large study examining the unmet health-related service needs of people aging with MS who are living in the Great Lakes region. For the purposes of this work, the Great Lakes Region includes the states of Minnesota, Wisconsin, Illinois, Indiana and Michigan. People aging with MS are defined as those individuals who are 45 years and older, while older adults with MS are considered to be age 60 and over.

LITERATURE REVIEW

The general concept of need is familiar to both clinicians and researchers, although formal definitions vary significantly. Overall, need is typically viewed as a gap between present circumstance and what is necessary or desired (Reviere, Berkowitz, Carter, & Ferguson, 1996; Witkin & Altschuld, 1995). Implicit in this definition is that unmet needs occur when gaps are not filled, which can be the consequence of unavailable services or supports, or ones that are available, but inaccessible due to physical, social or financial barriers.

There are a number of types of need that have been identified in the literature. Bradshaw's (1972) classic typology distinguishes felt need (want), expressed need (demand), comparative need (need based on comparisons to and equity with others), and normative need (expert definitions). It is this latter definition that is most commonly used in the individual assessment and treatment process in health care facilities, as well as in many community-based public health efforts. Often, the term "need" is linked to other descriptors in order to focus assessment and measurement efforts. For example, the current study focused on health-related service needs.

To date, research that has examined health-related service needs among people with MS have primarily focused on expressed needs (demands) and on normative needs (Bennett, Hamilton, Neutel, Pearson, & Talbot, 1977; Black, Grant, Lapsley, & Rawson, 1994; Freeman & Thompson, 2000; Kersten et al., 2000; Kersten & McLellan, 1995; Kraft, Freal, & Coryell, 1986; Somerset, Campbell, Sharp, & Peters, 2001; Stolp-Smith, 1998). The measurement of normative needs in these studies is typically achieved through a two-step process. Extent of symptoms and functional limitations are evaluated, and then these results are compared either to the health-related services that are available, the criteria for receipt of particular services, or the services that are actually received (Andrews & Henderson, 2000; Carr & Wolfe, 1976; Mullersdorf & Soderback, 1998).

Using these approaches, the estimation of need reflects the proportion of people who either use or meet criteria for available services, but who do not receive them (Andrews & Henderson, 2000). Underlying these estimations is the assumption that *services* rather than some other form of support (e.g., a friend, a change in environment) are required to reduce the initial need. In other words, these approaches to measuring health-related service need tend to define it in the context of the solution itself (i.e., the service, for example, occupational therapy) rather than the underlying issue or goal (e.g., improve employability) (Witkin & Altschuld, 1995). Fundamentally, normative approaches to measuring need, particularly in the health care sector, are philosophically based in a medical model system.

An additional critique of using a normative approach to defining and measuring need is that the perspectives of the persons under study are not directly considered and incorporated into the measurement process. Across the seven studies that explicitly explore the health-related needs of adults with MS (Bennett et al., 1977; Black et al., 1994; Freeman & Thompson, 2000; Kersten et al., 2000; Kraft et al., 1986; Somerset et al., 2001; Stolp-Smith, 1998), only one discussed incorporating the perspectives of people with MS in the development of the data collection instrument (Somerset et al., 2001). This limitation is important to consider when reviewing the findings of these studies, through which adults with MS have been found to have unmet health-related needs ranging from exercise advice and diet, to more specific topics such as obtaining information about new MS medications and how to manage urinary problems. Freeman and Thompson (2000) found that an important unmet health-related need among members of their sample was better and more flexible coordination of care in order to accommodate changes in their symptoms and abilities. Unfortunately, none of the existing needs assessment studies of persons with MS identified here have conducted analyses examining whether there are differences in needs between older and younger persons with MS.

Like the needs assessment research, studies examining the actual use of health-related services among persons with MS tend not to address age-related differences (Carton, Loos, Pacolet, Versieck & Vlietinck, 1998; Finlayson & DalMonte, 2002; Moorer, Surrmeijer & Zwanikken, 2000; Stolp-Smith, Atkinson, Campion, O'Brien & Rodriquez, 1998). One exception is the work by Finlayson and DalMonte (2002). These researchers found that age did not have a significant influence of the likelihood that a person with MS would see an occupational therapist, either in the past year or since diagnosis. In other health services utilization work, Stolp-Smith et al. (1998) found that younger people with MS use a broader range of health care services compared to younger people without MS. In addition, they found that older people with MS were less likely to use services related to cardiovascular care compared to their same age peers without MS. This finding is consistent with the work of Fleming and Blake (1994), who found that older adults with MS were less likely than their age and sex matched peers to be in the hospital for heart attack or failure, angina, cerebrovascular disease, diabetes or lung disease.

With the combination of the progressive nature of MS and normal life course changes due to age, it could be expected that older adults with MS may have perspectives on health-related services and associated needs that are different from those identified in these previous MS studies. Given this assumption, and the importance of client-centered perspectives for occupational therapy practice and research, this study began the process of identifying the health-related service needs among older adults with MS by talking to people most affected by the disease: People aging with MS, their family members, and their health care providers. Client-centered approaches require the involvement of the client (whether an individual or a collective) in identifying problems and potential solutions (Law, 1998). The specific questions that are addressed include:

1. How do people affected by MS interpret the term "health-related services?" What do they include under this rubric?
2. What images do people affected by MS hold of an older adult with a long-term diagnosis of MS (i.e., at least 20 years)?
3. Based on these images, what health-related services do people affected by MS feel older adults with MS need?
4. What factors do people affected by MS feel influence the actual utilization of health-related services by older adults with MS?

DESIGN AND METHODS

This study is the first phase of a large scale needs assessment that is seeking to identify the unmet health-related service needs among people aging with MS in the Great Lakes Region. The study is divided into three major phases: Focus groups with persons affected by MS (5 groups that included people with MS and family members; two groups of health care providers), telephone interviews with older adults with MS, and telephone interviews with informal caregivers (i.e., unpaid family members or friends) of older adults with MS.

The primary purpose of the focus group phase of the study was to identify critical health-related service issues facing older adults with MS and their caregivers (both formal and informal), and their greatest health-related service needs. Findings from this phase of the study will be used to modify and refine the telephone interview guides for phases two and three. Since this paper focuses solely on the first phase of the study, only it will be presented in the remainder of this methods description.

Sample

Sixty-seven individuals were purposively recruited to participate in one of seven focus groups held across five states. Five of these groups included only persons with MS or their family members (one in each of the participating states), while the other two groups included health care professionals serving persons with MS (Indiana and Minnesota). The decision to complete the health care professional focus groups in these two states was a function of time (due to traveling), budget constraints, and access to space to conduct the groups.

For all groups, we specifically sought participants who had a special interest in or expertise about aging with MS, either because of personal, professional, volunteer or family-related experiences. For example, we sought people with MS who were older themselves (i.e., over 60), and family members who provided assistance to older adults with MS. We also sought people with MS who volunteered in the Information and Referral area of the National Multiple Sclerosis Society (NMSS) chapters, even if they were not over 60 themselves. These individuals have a unique perspective on aging with MS because they are growing older with the disease themselves, and they have extensive knowledge of the types of issues and concerns other people with MS have about aging because of their volunteer role.

All participants were identified through NMSS staff members in the five states or through the members of the Study Advisory Group, which is made up of older adults with MS, family members of people with MS, and people associated with the NMSS in the Midwest (e.g., support group leaders, committee volunteers, program staff). The recruitment process involved having the Study Advisory Group member or the NMSS staff person contact a potential participant, give him/her a brief explanation of the focus groups (standard information was provided), and ask if he/she was willing to be contacted by a member of the study staff. The second author made a follow-up contact with the individual, if permission was granted. During this contact, a more detailed explanation of the study was provided, including an explanation of the focus groups and how they fit into the larger study. In addition, specific information about the time and place of the focus group and about the informed consent process was given.

In total, 67 individuals were contacted about participating in the focus groups, with 54 of these contacts occurring with people with MS or their family members. The remaining contacts (n = 13) were with health care professionals. Across these 67 contacts, 6 individuals did not respond to messages left for them (4 of these were health care professionals), 6 individuals declined to participate due to other commitments (all people with MS or family members), and 4 agreed to participate but did not show up for their scheduled focus group (all people with MS or family members). Consequently, fifty-one of the original 67 people contacted actually participated in one of the seven focus groups (participation rate = 76%). Table 1 provides a summary of the key characteristics of the focus group participants. Across the 34 people with MS, 3 were under 49 years of age, 17 were between 50 and 59 years of age, and 13 were over 60 years of age. One person did not report age. Unfortunately, no occupational therapists participated in the health professional groups either because of scheduling conflicts or lack of willingness to participate.

Instrumentation and Procedures

A semi-structured interview guide developed specifically for this study was used during the focus groups. It contained a series of open-ended questions and probes that were developed by the first author. Based on review and feedback by the members of the Study Advisory Group, revisions to the wording and ordering of the questions were made. The format of the interview guide allowed the same basic information to be collected across all groups, yet the open-ended format of the questions, together with the probes, allowed related but unanticipated issues and topics to emerge during the interviews (Krueger & Casey, 2000). Examples of questions that were used during the focus groups include: When you hear the term "health-related services" what services do you think of? When you think of a person who is over the age of 70 and has had MS for at least 20 years, what images come to your mind? Based on these images, what do you think are the health-related services that are needed by older adults with MS? What are some of the factors that you think explain or contribute to any variability in service utilization among older adults with MS?

Each group was facilitated by the first author, and co-facilitated by the second author. Both of the health care professional focus groups were restricted to one hour in length, while the focus groups for persons

TABLE 1. Participant Characteristics

	PwMS & Family (n = 42)	HCP (n = 9)	Total (n = 51)
Age			
Mean	59.0 years	47.5 years	57.0 years
Range	39-80	40-56	39-80
Sex (count)			
Female	25	8	33
Male	17	1	18
Connection to MS[1] (count)			
Person with MS	34	0	34
Family Member	11	0	18
Health Care Provider[2]	3	9	12
MS Society Volunteer	19	0	19
MS Society Staff	0	1	1
State (count)			
Illinois	6	0	6
Indiana	7	3	10
Michigan	8	0	8
Minnesota	12	6	18
Wisconsin	9	0	9

PwMS = People with MS
HCP = health care professionals
[1] - The numbers in the Connection to MS category do not match the total number of participants because some participants fit into more than one category. 43 participants reported dual roles, the most common of which was being a person with MS and a volunteer with the MS Society.
[2] - Health care professions represented: nursing (2), medicine (2), physical therapy (1), chaplain services (1), social work (3), psychology (1), therapeutic recreation (1) and mobility consultant (1).

with MS and their family members were limited to two hours in length. The difference in the group duration was a function of conducting the groups during the working hours of the health care professionals.

All groups began with introductions, an explanation of group rules, and a review and explanation of the informed consent process. Each focus group was audio-taped, and notes were taken on flipchart paper during the course of the groups. For three of the groups, the notes were comprehensive, and captured the contents of the discussion well. For the remaining 4 groups, the discussions were such that the bullet point format of the notes was unable to capture some of the most interesting contents of the discussions. For these groups, the audiotapes were also fully transcribed to aid in the analysis process.

Analysis

Since the majority of the questions asked during the focus groups required participants to generate lists of items (e.g., health-related services, images of older adults with MS, sources of utilization variability), a content analysis approach was used for this study (Miles & Huberman, 1994). The first step in the analysis was to combine each of the lists for each of the questions across all of the groups. The items on each list were then reviewed and those items that reflected the same or similar concepts were combined, for example, eye doctor and ophthalmologist. The second step in the analysis was to combine items into categories. This process involved the authors working independently to categorize the items on each of the lists, and then meeting to compare and discuss the categorizations. When there was disagreement, discussions were held until consensus was reached on categorizations, as well as the labels for the categories. Findings were summarized in table format using counts to display the data.

RESULTS

Interpretation of Health-Related Services

The first question that was asked during the focus groups was "When you hear the term 'health-related services' what services to you think of?" The lists generated by the groups were diverse in both content and length, but overall some common items emerged. As Table 2 shows, all groups identified physicians and transportation services under this rubric. Within the physician category, responses included general practitioners, neurologists, and urologists. It is interesting to note that transportation services were identified more often than many medically related services, including rehabilitation and home care. In addition to the items listed on Table 2, examples of other service categories identified by three or fewer of the groups included: Dental services, eye care, domestic violence services, alternative services (e.g., acupuncture, massage), home maintenance programs, end-of-life services (e.g., funeral arrangements), health insurance, and employment services.

TABLE 2. Interpretation of "Health-Related Services"

Most common items included as "health-related services"	PwMS & Family (n = 5 groups)	HCP (n = 2 groups)	Total (n = 7 groups)
Physicians	5	2	7
Transportation & community accessibility	5	2	7
Pharmaceutical services	5	1	6
Exercise & physical wellness services	5	1	6
Nutrition & meals on wheels programs	5	1	6
Information and referral services	5	1	6
Emergency medical care services	5	1	6
Formal case management and coordination	4	2	6
Mental health services	4	2	6
Financial services and support	4	2	6
Traditional rehabilitation services	5	0	5
Assistive technology services	5	0	5
Social well-being services	5	0	5
Peer lead support services	4	1	5
Professional home care services	4	1	5
Housing services	4	1	5
Advocacy and legal services	4	0	4
Family and caregiver services	3	1	4
Spirituality services	2	2	4

PwMS = People with MS
HCP = Health Care Professionals

Image of Older Adults with MS

Both groups of participants (i.e., persons with MS and family members; health care professionals) had difficulty responding to the question, "When you think of a person who is over the age of 70 and has had MS for at least 20 years, what images come to your mind?" This difficulty stemmed from the fact that participants identified their images as varying widely depending on the type of MS an individual has and whether the person is male or female (participants noted that men with MS typically progress in the disease more quickly than women). Ultimately, the images generated in each group followed a continuum from someone who was extremely limited in their abilities, to someone who was functioning well within his/her roles and environment.

At the one end of the continuum, participants described an older adult with a long-term diagnosis of MS as someone who is having difficulty with mobility (using a walker or wheelchair), is experiencing declining cognitive abilities, and whose mental health is deteriorating. In addition, they described this person as experiencing increasing MS-related symptoms and consequences, for example, more fatigue and bladder infections. Some groups identified that an older adult with MS may be bedridden, and in need of personal care and/or supervision. Participants felt that such an individual would most likely be eating poorly, have functional limitations, and require assistive technology for everyday activities. Overall, at this end of the image continuum, participants described an older adult with MS as being depressed, isolated, experiencing decreased quality of life, and having a questionable will to live. This person would lack recent information regarding MS and would have a very stressed caregiver.

At the opposite end of the image continuum, participants described an older adult with a long-term diagnosis of MS as someone who is living independently in a modified and convenient home, is utilizing available resources, is working hard, and is walking, driving and traveling with the use of assistive technology. Participants described this individual as having a lot of experience and knowledge about MS, and as someone who has the ability to learn and adapt to changes in his/her life and disease. Overall, at this end of the image continuum, participants described this older adult with MS as being a vital individual, who wants to make a difference in the world and who has come to terms with having MS. This older adult with MS has continued to perform previous life roles.

Health-Related Service Needs of Older Adults with MS

After generating their images of an older adult with MS, focus group participants were asked "Based on these images, what do you think are the health-related services that are needed by older adults with MS?" While the lists of health-related services that were generated earlier in the focus groups was long and diverse, these lists were considerably shorter and more focused, both for the persons with MS and family members, as well as for the health care professionals.

Transportation was the only service identified by all seven focus groups as an important health-related service need among older adults with MS. Among the five groups made up of persons with MS and their family members, the other health-related service needs that were most frequently identified included housing, professional home care, social well-being programs, pharmaceutical services, nutrition programs, and exercise, wellness and physical well-being services. One of these focus groups also talked about the need for a family member or "overseer"; someone who could manage and coordinate their care, including doctor's appointments, medications, and other programs and services such as insurance and financial paperwork. In comparison, both health care professional groups identified case management and financial services as important health-related service needs. See Table 3.

One of the important differences between the health-related service needs expressed by the persons with MS and their family members and those identified by the health care professionals was the qualifiers that were placed on the services. For example, in the responses given by per-

TABLE 3. Health-Related Needs

Most common items included as "health-related needs"	PwMS & Family (n = 5 groups)	HCP (n = 2 groups)	Total (n = 7 groups)
Physicians	1	1	2
Transportation & community accessibility	5	2	7
Pharmaceutical services	3	0	3
Exercise & physical wellness services	3	1	4
Nutrition & meals on wheels programs	3	0	3
Information and referral services	1	0	1
Emergency medical care services	2	1	3
Formal case management and coordination	0	2	2
Mental health services	2	1	3
Financial services and support	2	2	4
Traditional rehabilitation services	1	0	1
Assistive technology services	2	0	2
Social well-being services	3	0	3
Peer lead support services	1	0	1
Professional home care services	3	1	4
Housing services	4	0	4
Advocacy and legal services	2	0	2
Family and caregiver services	0	1	1
Spirituality services	0	1	1

PwMS = People with MS
HCP = Health Care Professionals

sons with MS and their family members it was common for us to hear adjectives such as "good quality," "compassionate," "knowledgeable," "well-trained," "respectful," or "affordable" in the process of naming a particular type of service or service provider. In comparison, the participants in the health care professional groups tended to simply identify the service or service provider. In other words, for the persons with MS and their family members, their health-related service needs were not for just a particular skill or knowledge set that the service or service provider offered, but rather for this set in combination with particular characteristics of the service delivery process.

Factors Influencing Utilization

After having the focus group participants discuss health-related services, their images of an older adult with MS, and what the needs of such a person might be, we asked each group: "What factors do you think contribute to whether an older adult will use these [needed] services or not?" Participants' responses ranged from health status factors, to features and characteristics of the service, to social support factors and personal skills. See Table 4.

Factors related to health status, and physical or disease characteristics were the most commonly identified ones that participants felt would influence whether an older adult with MS would choose to use a needed health-related service. Participants felt that people with more disabilities or poorer health status would be more likely to seek service use. They also felt that women, in general, were more likely to seek services than men. All seven focus groups discussed at least one or two items within this category of influencing factors.

A second group of influencing factors that were identified by participants was labeled *personal skills, education and knowledge.* Within this grouping, participants discussed how one's knowledge of available services, knowing how to "work the system" and knowing how to complete the necessary paperwork all enabled older adults with MS to use health-related services. One's ability to self-assess his/her health-related needs was also identified by participants, but this was a factor that was identified as potentially being a facilitator of service utilization (i.e., recognize a need and seek a service) as well as a barrier to utilization (i.e., do not recognize a need). All of the focus groups that included persons with MS and their family members discussed at least one or two items within this category; neither of the health care professional groups identified this area.

TABLE 4. Factors Contributing to Variability in Service Use Among Older Adults with MS

Category	Key examples from the Focus Groups
Health Status/Physical Characteristics/Disease	Type of MS
	Level of Health
	Extent of disability
	Sex
	Cognitive issues
Personal Skills/Knowledge/Education	Knowledge of available services
	Knowing how to complete the paperwork
	Ability to self-evaluate needs
	Knowing how to "work the system"
Social Support/Social Factors	Extent of support (family, community)
	Availability of assistance for paperwork
	Access to personal service recommendations
	Extent of social isolation
Financial resources and time	Insurance coverage
	Money
	Time
Service Characteristics	Access point (e.g., physician, MS Society)
	Knowledge of providers
	Convenience/inconvenience of service
	Location, distance and transportation
	Accessibility
Personal Traits & Characteristics	Attitude and mood
	Persistence and stubbornness
	Extent of acceptance or denial of problems
	Extent of initiative and sense of control
	Extent of personal crisis
	Extent of personal pride

Social supports and factors related to the social environment were identified by six of the focus groups as influencing the health-related service utilization of an older adult with MS. Having a supportive family that was close by, as well as having supportive friends and neighbors were identified as increasing the probability that a person would use a health-related service. Participants felt that strong social supports would suggest helpful services, help people access these services (e.g., help with transportation, completing paperwork), and generally encourage service use that may enable the person with MS to complete necessary and desired activities. Alternatively, participants felt that a person who was socially isolated may be less likely to use services because he/she may not have access to information and personal referrals for specific services.

An additional area that participants identified as contributing to the variability in utilization of health-related services was the features and characteristics of the service itself. This category was discussed in six of the seven focus groups. Participants discussed how proximity, ease of physical access, and general convenience facilitated the use of health-related services. Services that involved lengthy commutes, inaccessible parking and complicated paperwork were going to discourage utilization. Cost of services was also identified by participants, but in the context of access to personal financial resources. Having money and insurance were identified as facilitating health-related service use by one of the health care professional groups, and four of the groups made up of persons with MS and family members.

The final category of factors influencing health-related service use that was identified by focus group participants was labeled personal traits and characteristics. Having a positive attitude, being accepting of functional and health limitations, and taking initiative to control one's circumstance were identified as increasing the probability that an older adult with MS would use a health-related service. Hitting a crisis point in one's life (e.g., sudden deterioration in health, loss of a support person, deterioration in mobility status, etc.) would also likely increase the chances of utilization. Alternatively, being depressed, being stubborn, and having a strong sense of pride (i.e., unwilling to accept help) were felt to decrease the chances of utilization. All of the focus groups noted at least one factor within this category of influencers.

DISCUSSION

This paper has presented the findings from the first phase of a large study examining the unmet health-related service needs of older adults with MS and their family members. In this context, the purpose of the focus groups was to identify critical health-related service issues and needs in order to incorporate this information into the development and refinement of the data collection tools for phases two (i.e., telephone interviews with older adults with MS) and three (i.e., telephone interviews with caregivers of older adults with MS) of the overall study. Findings from the focus groups have provided insights into specific questions that need to be included in the telephone interviews, as well as ways of wording these questions.

More generally, the findings of the focus group phase show that participants, particularly those with MS and their family members, viewed health-related services very broadly and included services oriented towards health promotion (both physical and social), community accessibility, and support to remain at home. In comparison, health care professionals tended to focus more on medically related services and the coordination of the different components of the health care sector, as well as the professionals working within this sector. Many other researchers, in the MS field as well as others, have found differences in perspectives on needs between health professionals and their clients (Rothwell, McDowell, Wong & Dorman, 1997). These differences highlight the critical importance of utilizing a client-centered approach in occupational therapy practice to ensure that our interactions and interventions with clients are addressing what they identify as most important. Of particular interest for client-centered practice is the emphasis that persons with MS and their family members placed on the quality, accessibility, compassion and knowledge of service providers.

Transportation was one area of consistency across all of the focus groups, both in terms of identifying health-related services as well as needs. All groups emphasized the important role of accessible transportation in terms of accessing services and people, and meeting other health-related needs. While occupational therapists provide driving-related assessments and interventions, the emphasis on transportation systems and services in these focus groups point to our need to be more involved in broader system-level advocacy regarding accessible transportation, together with our clients and professional colleagues.

In our findings, it is interesting to note that both persons with MS and family members, as well as health care professionals, identified the importance of care coordination. This finding is consistent with the work of Freeman and Thompson (2000). The key difference across our groups was in the nature of this coordination, and who was felt to be the most appropriate person to fulfill this role. Persons with MS and their family members emphasized that this role was an informal one that was most appropriately filled within the family or immediate social network. In addition, they viewed the role more broadly in terms of the potential tasks that may be performed. The health care professionals tended to view this role as a formal one focused primarily on medically-related issues. Regardless of this difference, both groups emphasized that this role and need was long term in nature. For occupational therapists, these findings suggest that we need to actively involve family members in our work with persons with MS so that they can fulfill the role as care coordinator, or alternatively, we actively seek this role for ourselves within the context of our regular practice in the care system.

Across our groups, services focusing on health promotion, both for physical and social health, were identified as being an important component of health related services. In terms of needs, the groups made up of persons with MS and family members emphasized these types of needs to a greater extent than health care professionals. In previous work by Somerset et al. (2001), diet and exercise advice were found to be important needs of adults with MS, and our participants mentioned both of these areas. Nevertheless, only the groups made up of persons with MS and family members identified nutrition-related services as an important need in the current study. Overall, the identification of health promotion needs during the focus groups suggests important potential roles for occupational therapists with older adults with MS, and points to opportunities to use our existing knowledge of falls prevention, home safety, and occupation for health with this population.

Across the groups, only the persons with MS and family members emphasized social well-being needs, in particular, the need for socialization, companionship, encouragement and support. Furthermore, they discussed the important role that a strong support network had in discovering and facilitating access to health-related services, particularly those that were outside of the traditional medical system. It is interesting that our participants identified and focused on these socialization needs and roles, particularly given their existing linkages with the National Multiple Sclerosis Society, and its programs and supports. It is unclear the extent to which this need might be greater among people without these linkages. Our ability to understand this need is limited by our active, articulate and socially engaged participants. Overall, we found our findings regarding social well-being to be consistent with the findings of Kersten et al. (2000), who identified self-actualization (i.e., activities that enable a person to be socially and intellectually fulfilled) to be an important unmet need of persons with MS. These findings further point to the critical need for a client-centered approach to working with persons with MS. Without such an approach it is feasible that these types of broader social needs would not be addressed in assessment or intervention.

Exercise and physical well-being needs were emphasized strongly by our participants. One focus group discussed the importance of preventative physical therapy services, and the need for physical therapy that goes beyond the acute, exacerbation phases of MS. Of interest is the fact that none of the groups identified a need for occupational therapy services, although many of the outcomes that an occupational therapist might work towards with a client were discussed at length (e.g., accessible housing, community accessibility, personal advocacy, social well-being). This observation reinforces a common feeling among occupational therapists: While potential clients may value the outcomes of occupational therapy intervention, these same individuals are unclear about who we are and what we do. In other words, they may be able to identify their needs, but do not recognize that an occupational therapist could work with them to address these needs. This finding points to a problem in occupational therapy's professional public relations and communications.

In the context of discussing physical health needs, one of the focus groups identified the challenges of obtaining age-related preventative tests (e.g., mammograms, colonostomy) due to the inaccessibility of many doctors' offices, as well as their examining tables or diagnostic machines. The insight gained through this discussion was the extent of influence and interaction that occurs across many of the unmet health-related service needs identified by participants. In particular, transportation and community accessibility were discussed as barriers to being able to meet many other health-related service needs. This challenge was particularly emphasized in the focus groups held in Indiana (both groups) and Wisconsin, where a number of participants were from more rural areas of the state, or alternatively, had contact with individuals in these less-serviced areas. In other MS needs assessment research, geographical differences in needs have been identified among persons with MS (Bennett et al., 1977; Black et al., 1994; Kraft et al., 1986). These differences point to the importance of exploring geographical variability in needs more closely. In addition, they once again point to the need for occupational therapists to be more involved in broader social action and advocacy efforts to ensure equitable access to services among our current and potential clients.

Accessibility issues were also reflected in the discussions about the importance of accessibility within the home. Participants, particularly those with MS and their family members, talked about the challenges of finding accessible and affordable housing that could meet their changing physical assistance needs. Black et al. (1994), Freeman and Thompson (2000) and Kraft et al. (1986) have previously raised problems of accessibility in their findings. A key difference between our findings and the findings of other authors was that our participants (those with MS and their family members) took the accessibility discussions to a higher level. That is, rather than simply identifying the need for community and home accessibility, they emphasized that changes to accessibility were not going to happen without strong advocacy efforts, enforcement of the Americans with Disabilities Act, and better and more knowledgeable professionals who could provide information and consultation about accessibility options for persons with a disability. Occupational therapists have a responsibility to ensure we are meeting this call.

The differences identified between the groups of persons with MS and family members compared to the health care professionals may be the consequence of a number of factors. It may be a function of the types of health care professionals participating in our groups (i.e., their disciplinary foci), the limited time we had available to explore and probe some of their ideas, or the types of clients they saw (e.g., more disabled than the people in our other focus groups). Alternatively, they may have held a different perspective on need than the persons with MS and their family members. In general, other published research has shown dramatic differences in the viewpoints of health professionals and their clients regarding needs and appropriate interventions (Rothwell et al., 1997), and our study may simply be consistent with this other work.

Overall, this study is limited by its use of key informants, all of whom were very knowledgeable about existing services and appeared to be able to find and get the services that they needed or wanted. At the same time, their multiple roles (e.g., person with MS and volunteer; family member and health care professional; etc.) provided unique insights that benefited this research effort. An additional limitation was our inability to conduct focus groups in geographically diverse areas and to discuss differences in the health-related services needs by age. This study does not indicate whether the needs identified are also experienced by younger people with MS. Future research would benefit from addressing these limitations in order to expand our understanding of the needs of older adults with MS, and people aging with the disease.

CONCLUSION

This paper has presented the findings from the first phase of a large study examining the unmet health-related service needs of older adults with MS and their caregivers. Through the use of focus groups with people affected by MS, we found that health-related services are viewed very broadly. Based on very diverse images of older adults with MS, health-related service needs focused on the areas of health promotion (both physical and social), community accessibility, and support to remain at home. Transportation was the most commonly identified unmet health-related service need.

Persons with MS and family members emphasized the necessity of having health-care professionals who are knowledgeable and well trained about MS and its associated challenges and implications, and who are compassionate and caring towards their experiences living with MS. This challenges occupational therapists in all roles: Educators to be comprehensive, practitioners to be client-centered, and researchers to include the perspectives of people affected by the disease.

REFERENCES

Andrews, G., & Henderson, S. (2000). *Unmet needs in psychiatry: Problems, resources, responses.* Cambridge, UK: Cambridge University Press.

Bennett, L., Hamilton, R., Neutel, C. I., Pearson, J. C., & Talbot, B. (1977). Survey of persons with multiple sclerosis in Ottawa, 1974-75. *Canadian Journal of Public Health, 68* (2), 141-147.

Black, D. A., Grant, C., Lapsley, H. M., & Rawson, G. K. (1994). The services and social needs of people with multiple sclerosis in New South Wales, Australia. *Journal of Rehabilitation, 60*(4), 60-65.

Bradshaw, J. L. (1972). A taxonomy of social need. In G.McLachlan (Ed.), *Problems and progress in medical care: Essays on current research* (pp. 71-82). London: Oxford University Press.

Carr, W., & Wolfe, S. (1976). Unmet needs as sociomedical indicators. *International Journal of Health Services, 6*(3), 417-430.

Carton, H., Loos, R., Pacolet, J., Versieck, K., & Vlietinck, R. (1998). Utilisation and cost of professional care and assistance according to disability of patients with multiple sclerosis in Flanders (Belgium). *Journal of Neurology, Neurosurgery and Psychiatry, 64*(4), 444-450.

Finlayson, M., & Dalmonte, J. (2002). Predicting the use of occupational therapy among people with multiple sclerosis in Atlantic Canada. *Canadian Journal of Occupational Therapy, 69* (4), 239-248

Fleming, S.T., & Blake, R.L. (1994). Patterns of comorbidity in elderly patients with multiple sclerosis. *Journal of Clinical Epidemiology, 47* (10), 1127-1132.

Freeman, J. A., & Thompson, A. J. (2000). Community services in multiple sclerosis: Still a matter of chance. *Journal of Neurology, Neurosurgery & Psychiatry, 69*(6), 728-732.

Kersten, P., & McLellan, D. L. (1995). The assessment of need in multiple sclerosis. *MS Management, 2,* 50-54.

Kersten, P., McLellan, D. L., Gross-Paju, K., Grigoriadis, N., Bencivenga, R., Beneton, C., Charlier, M., Ketelaer, P., & Thompson, A. J. (2000). A questionnaire assessment of unmet needs for rehabilitation services and resources for people with multiple sclerosis: Results of a pilot survey in five European countries. *Clinical Rehabilitation, 14*(1), 42-49.

Kraft, G. H., Freal, J. E., & Coryell, J. K. (1986). Disability, disease duration, and rehabilitation service needs in multiple sclerosis: Patient perspectives. *Archives of Physical Medicine & Rehabilitation, 67*(3), 164-168.

Krueger, R.A., & Casey, M.A. (2000). *Focus groups: A practical guide for applied research.* Third Edition. Thousand Oaks: Sage.

Miles, M.B., & Huberman, A.M. (1994). *Qualitative data analysis: An expanded sourcebook, 2nd edition.* Thousand Oaks, CA: Sage.

Miller, D.H., Hornabrook, R.W., & Purdie, G. (1992). The natural history of multiple sclerosis: A regional study with longitudinal data. *Journal of Neurology, Neurosurgery and Psychiatry, 55*(5), 341-346.

Moorer, P., Suurmeijer, T.H., & Zwanikken, C.P. (2000). Health care utilization by people with multiple sclerosis in The Netherlands: Results of two separate studies. *Disability and Rehabilitation, 22* (16), 695-701.

Mullersdorf, M. & Soderback, I. (1998). Needs assessment methods in healthcare and rehabilitation. *Critical Reviews in Physical & Rehabilitation Medicine, 10*(1), 57-73.

Law, M. (1998). *Client-centered occupational therapy.* Thorofare, NJ: Slack, Inc.

Reviere, R., Berkowitz, S., Carter, C. C., & Ferguson, C. G. (1996). Introduction: Setting the stage. In R. Reviere, S. Berkowitz, C.C. Carter, & C.G. Ferguson (Eds). *Needs assessment: A creative and practical guide for social scientists.* (pp. 1-14). Washington, DC: Taylor & Francis.

Rothwell, P.M., McDowell, Z., Wong, C.K., & Dorman, P.J. (1997). Doctors and patients don't agree: Cross sectional study of patients' and doctors' perceptions and assessments of disability in multiple sclerosis. *British Medical Journal, 314,* 1580-1583.

Somerset, M., Campbell, R., Sharp, D. J., & Peters, T. J. (2001). What do people with MS want and expect from health care services? *Health Expectations, 4*(1), 29-37.

Stolp-Smith, K.A. (1998). Lifetime care needs of individuals with multiple sclerosis. *Journal of Spinal Cord Medicine, 21*(2), 121-123.

Stolp-Smith, K., Atkinson, E. J., Campion, M. E., O'Brien, P.C., & Rodriguez, M. (1998). Health care utilization in multiple sclerosis: A population-based study in Olmsted County, MN. *Neurology, 50*(6), 1594-1600.

Weinshenker, B. G. (1995). The natural history of multiple sclerosis. *Neurological Clinics of North America, 13*(1), 119-146.

Witkin, B.R., & Altschuld, J.W. (1995). *Planning and conducting needs assessments: A practical guide.* Thousand Oaks: Sage.

Analysis of Symptoms, Functional Impairments, and Participation in Occupational Therapy for Individuals with Multiple Sclerosis

Letha J. Mosley, MEd, OTR/L
Gregory P. Lee, PhD
Mary L. Hughes, MD
Charlotte Chatto, PT, MS

SUMMARY. The aim of this study was to identify client factors that may influence physicians' decision to refer individuals with multiple sclerosis (MS) to occupational therapy (OT). Study participants were

---

Letha J. Mosley is a PhD student, University of Georgia (E-mail: lethaj@uga.edu). She was Assistant Professor, Department of Occupational Therapy, Medical College of Georgia, at the time of this study.

Gregory P. Lee is Professor, Departments of Occupational Therapy and Neurology (EF-110), Medical College of Georgia, Augusta GA 30912 (E-mail: glee@mail.mcg.edu).

Mary L. Hughes is Assistant Professor, Department of Neurology, Medical College of Georgia, Augusta, GA 30912 (E-mail: MHughes@neur.INET).

Charlotte Chatto is Assistant Professor, Department of Physical Therapy (CH-100), Medical College of Georgia, Augusta, GA 30912 (E-mail: cchatto@mail.mcg.edu).

The authors gratefully acknowledge the assistance of Maria Poo Garcia in data collection, data management, and manuscript preparation.

This study was supported, in part, by a grant from Berlex Laboratories, Inc.

[Haworth co-indexing entry note]: "Analysis of Symptoms, Functional Impairments, and Participation in Occupational Therapy for Individuals with Multiple Sclerosis." Mosley, Letha J. et al. Co-published simultaneously in *Occupational Therapy in Health Care* (The Haworth Press, Inc.) Vol. 17, No. 3/4, 2003, pp. 27-43; and: *Occupational Therapy Practice and Research with Persons with Multiple Sclerosis* (ed: Marcia Finlayson) The Haworth Press, Inc., 2003, pp. 27-43. Single or multiple copies of this article are available for a fee from The Haworth Document Delivery Service [1-800-HAWORTH, 9:00 a.m. - 5:00 p.m. (EST). E-mail address: docdelivery@haworthpress.com].

10.1300/J003v17n03_03

seen in an MS clinic in which a physician referral was required prior to receipt of OT services. The symptoms and functional impairments of 40 individuals with MS who were either seen or not seen for OT services were compared. Findings show that individuals with MS who were referred to OT reported more difficulties with speaking or swallowing, hand tremors, uncontrolled urinary urgency, weakness of the legs, and performing functional activities than individuals with MS who did not receive OT services. Results also suggest that difficulties in functional mobility, work, community mobility and meal preparation were more likely to prompt OT referral and subsequent therapy for individuals who had attended the MS Clinic than any specific sign or symptom. *[Article copies available for a fee from The Haworth Document Delivery Service: 1-800-HAWORTH. E-mail address: <docdelivery@haworthpress.com> Website: <http://www.HaworthPress.com> © 2003 by The Haworth Press, Inc. All rights reserved.]*

KEYWORDS. Occupational therapy, multiple sclerosis, functional impairments, activities of daily living, areas of occupation, referral, participation

INTRODUCTION

Multiple sclerosis (MS) is a debilitating neurological disorder in which the oligodendrocytes that form myelin sheaths along the axon of neurons in the central nervous system are destroyed (Paty & Ebers, 1998). This deteriorating disorder has a variable and unpredictable course of progression, including patterns of remission and relapse with varying signs and symptoms that can negatively influence independence and quality of life (Somerset, Sharp & Campbell, 2002). With an average age of onset of 30 years, individuals with MS may have a relatively normal, or in atypical cases, a slightly shorter life expectancy (Paty & Ebers, 1998).

Purpose

Given the average age of onset, life expectancy, and impairments that may interfere with the independence and quality of life of persons with MS, it is important for health care providers to make timely referrals for services that may be of benefit. Occupational therapy (OT) has been used successfully to diminish or slow down the advancement of underlying impairments and sustain or improve the function for persons with MS (Mathiowetz, Matuska & Murphy, 2001; Gillen, 2002; Baker & Tickle-Degnen, 2001). Typically, in the medical model of practice in the United States a physician referral is necessary for occupational therapy evaluation, intervention, and reimbursement of services. Physician referrals made on the basis of an assessment of the individual often include objective data and subjective information collected during the evaluation process, however the factors that prompt physician referrals of persons with MS to OT have not been thoroughly researched and documented.

This study was conducted to determine if there were any significant differences in signs, symptoms, or functional difficulties of individuals with MS who were referred to and received occupational therapy services in comparison to those who did not receive a referral and subsequent services. The hypotheses in this study were:

1. individuals who are referred to and received occupational therapy will report more severe symptoms of MS than individuals who are not seen for OT services;
2. there will be differences in the symptoms of individuals seen for OT when compared with individuals not seen for OT; and
3. those individuals with MS who report functional difficulties will be referred to and receive OT more often than those individuals who report no functional difficulties.

By understanding this information, OT practitioners may be able to better advocate for individuals with MS to receive timely and appropriate referral for OT.

Client Factors Influenced by MS

As described within the *Occupational Therapy Practice Framework: Domain and Process* (Youngstrom et al., 2002), client factors include body functions and body structures that may influence performance in areas of occupation (AOC). Individuals with MS may present with impairments of these client factors, the most significant changes are in the visual, vestibular, sensory, and motor systems (Paty & Ebers, 1998). Typical signs and symptoms associated with MS include, but are not limited to, blurred or double vision, fatigue, decreased balance, and poor control of bowel and bladder. The most commonly identified symptom is fatigue (van den Noort & Holland, 1999). Clinical signs frequently documented include abnormal eye responses, localized weakness, and gait disorders.

In addition, physical problems such as ataxia, tremor, and sensory loss are frequently cited in the literature as influencing the functional independence of persons with MS. Additional problems related to inability to concentrate, loss of memory, depression, and euphoria may be just as devastating for individuals with this condition. These impairments may negatively influence an individual's ability to safely, independently and efficiently perform AOCs such as activities of daily living (ADLs), instrumental ADLs (IADLs), education, work, and social participation (Amato et al., 1995; Dyck & Jongbloed, 2000; Gulick, 1998; Somerset, Sharp & Campbell, 2002).

Interventions to Address Impaired Client Factors and Function

Interventions to prevent or slow down the debilitating effects of MS over a person's lifetime may be provided in the community, inpatient rehabilitation, or on an outpatient basis. These services may include but are not limited to occupational therapy, physical therapy, speech and language pathology, neuropsychology, and nursing services (Freeman et al. 1997; Freeman & Thompson, 2000). Rehabilitation has been found to reduce the level of disability and handicap in individuals with MS despite the progressive nature of the underlying impairments that influence function (Freeman et al., 1997).

Several studies have evaluated the efficacy of treatments that are employed by occupational therapists to sustain function and quality of life. Mathiowetz et al. (2001) found strong evidence that a specific program of education for energy conservation among persons with MS who had a primary problem of fatigue had a positive impact on cognitive, physical, and social functions after the instructional intervention. Individual gains were sustained for at least six weeks after completion of the educational activity. Gillen (2002), using a task-oriented approach, demonstrated in a case study the ability of occupational therapy intervention to improve the functional mobility of a client with multiple sclerosis. After specific interventions the person improved from a level of 'minimal assistance' to 'independent with extra time and equipment' in spite of continuing deficits of tremors and incoordination. Wellness and rehabilitation interventions implemented by occupational therapy have also been reported, in a consumer magazine, to improve or delay a decline in health status among individuals with MS (Lou, Classen, & Peirce, 2002).

In a meta-analysis of the effectiveness of physical, psychological, and functional interventions in treating clients with multiple sclerosis, Baker and Tickle-Degnen (2001) found that occupational therapy related treatments had a strong positive effect on the effects of MS. The 23 studies reviewed suggested OT related interventions were moderately effective in enhancing the lives of individuals with MS. Seventy-six percent of individuals with MS who had therapy had positive results while only 24% of clients exhibited positive results without therapy, suggesting a large and positive effect of therapeutic interventions on outcomes.

To compensate for various neurological impairments and increase safety in the home, individuals with MS may be evaluated and trained in the use of assistive devices (AD). In a survey of 427 people diagnosed with MS in Atlantic Canada, Finlayson, Guglielmello and Liefer (2001) determined the average number of AD in the possession of individuals with MS was 3.4. The likelihood of having AD was increased by several factors, one of which was having an occupational therapist. Although the study does not specify the time at which these devices are introduced, the person's severity level may have influenced the number of AD acquired.

Current Trends in the Use of Occupational Therapy

Little research has been conducted on referral trends for OT in the treatment of MS, particularly in the United States. In the United Kingdom, Freeman and Thompson (2000) surveyed 150 adults with MS and found 21% of the 150 received OT, but of those individuals identified as severely disabled 41% were seen by OT. These results showed that the greater the level of symptom severity, the higher the percentage of individuals referred for OT services. In a survey on the use of alternative health therapies by individuals in southern New England with MS, only 19% indicated receiving OT services (Fawcett, Sidney, Hanson & Riley-Lawless, 1994). Finlayson and DalMonte (2002) reported that individuals with MS in Atlantic Canada who had more functional limitations, and who were seen by a greater number of health professionals, were more likely to be seen by an OT. The findings of these researchers brings into question whether, in the Canadian service system, OT may be viewed as a complimentary service versus a primary service for this population. In this same study, individuals with MS who had been hospitalized within the previous year were the most likely to be seen by an OT.

Occupational therapy referral has also been studied for persons with conditions other than MS. Soderback and Paulsson (1997) completed a study in which primary care nurses at a Swedish acute care cancer hospital assessed the need for occupational therapy by completing a questionnaire about their clients based on a list of interventions offered by occupational therapy. Of the 88 individuals included in the study, 26% had physician referrals to OT while 47% were judged by nursing to be in need of OT but had not been referred. There was a significant difference between expressed need for OT and the number of actual occupational therapy referrals. The questionnaire was newly developed; therefore, further investigation is required to substantiate the findings. In a survey of the College of Family Physicians of Canada regarding referrals to OT, 13.6% (72 of 529) of physician respondents referred individuals with early rheumatoid arthritis to OT, while during the later stages of the disease; the referral rate increased to 44.8% (Glazier et al., 1996). This indicates a tendency of physicians to refer to OT after symptoms become prominent enough to influence function rather than for primary prevention or wellness.

While little research has been documented on referral and participation in occupational therapy by individuals with MS in the United States, in other countries one consideration seems to be related to the severity of the disease process. The current study was designed to identify any significant signs, symptoms or functional impairments that prompted participation in OT in a medical system in which a referral is required prior to treatment.

METHOD

Participants

Seventy-nine individuals with MS who were receiving medical care at a specialty outpatient Neurology MS clinic located in a university medical center, and who also had a valid and current mailing address were sent a questionnaire. Of the 79 questionnaires mailed, 40 (51%) were returned. These 40 individuals served as the sample for this study, including thirty-one females and 9 males.

Survey Instrument

The investigators developed the questionnaire used in this study for a larger grant funded study approved by the institution's Human Assurance Committee. The investigators represented health care disciplines including occupational therapy, physical therapy, neurology, neuropsychology, and nursing. The purpose of the questionnaire was to primarily examine the symptoms, course of illness, treatment, degree of social support, and satisfaction with medical care among individuals with multiple sclerosis. The self-administered survey consisted of 73 multiple-choice questions. For the purposes of this study, three questions were utilized. The first question asked respondents to identify whether or not they were seen in occupational therapy. Responses to this item provided the basis for classifying participants into either the OT group or No OT group. A second question evaluated the presence and severity (if applicable) of 28 common MS symptoms on a four-point Likert-type scale (0 = none, 1 = mild, 2 = moderate, and 3 = severe). The third question asked respondents to indicate whether or not they were experiencing difficulties performing any of the following tasks related to areas of occupation and performance skills: Talking; bathing, hygiene and grooming; getting dressed; walking or getting around the house; cooking; driving; working; or other in which participants wrote in specific responses. Thirty-one (78%) of the 40 participants indicated difficulty in at least one Area of Occupation.

Data Analysis

Symptom severity differences between groups were examined using Mann-Whitney U test since the questionnaire data subjected to statistical analysis was ordinal. Alpha (probability) level was set at an *a priori* p-value of $\leq$ .05. Non-parametric Chi-square comparisons were used to evaluate whether there were significant differences in the frequency of functional impairments between the two groups. Demographic variables that were interval or ratio level data were analyzed using one-way analyses of variance. Statistical analyses were conducted using the Statview II statistical software package.

RESULTS

Description of Participants

Participants were classified into two groups based upon self-report to a survey question that asked whether or not they had seen an occupational therapist (OT). Twelve (30%) of the 40 individuals reported being seen by an OT (OT group), and 28 (70%) reported not being seen by an OT (No OT group).

Mean age of the OT group was 47.8 (standard deviation [sd] = 17.6) years. Mean educational attainment was 14.9 (sd = 2.9) years. Eleven (92%) were female and one (8%) was male. Nine (75%) individuals in the OT group were White and three (25%) were African-American. Ten (83%) individuals lived in the immediate vicinity of the hospital and were considered as having a "suburban" residence while two (17%) individuals had a rural residence. Socioeconomic status (SES) was determined using Hollinghead's (1957) two-factor index for social position. Hollinghead's five classes of social position were collapsed to form three SES groups. Lower class and lower middle class were combined to form one "lower" class group, and upper class was combined with upper middle class to form one "upper" class group. Within the OT group, there were three (25%) lower class, six (50%) middle class, and three (25%) upper class participants.

Mean age of the 28 individuals comprising the No OT group was 46.6 (sd = 10. 6) years. Mean educational attainment was 13.5 (sd = 3.0) years. Twenty (71%) were female and eight (29%) were male. Seventeen (61%) individuals in the No OT group were white and eleven (39%) were African-American. Seventeen individuals (61%) lived in the immediate vicinity of the hospital and were considered as having a "suburban" residence while eleven (39%) individuals had a rural residence. With regard to socioeconomic status (SES) in the No OT group, there were twelve (43%) lower class, twelve (43%) middle class, and four (14%) upper class participants.

There were no statistically significant differences between the OT and No OT groups with regard to age ($F = 0.078$, $df = 1, 38$, $p = .78$), years of education ($F = 1.87$, $df = 1, 38$, $p = .18$), gender (Chi-square = 1.97, $df = 1$, $p = .16$), race (Chi-square = 0.75, $df = 1$, $p = .38$), place of residence (Chi-square = 1.96, $df = 1$, $p = .16$), or socioeconomic status (Chi-square = 1.36, $df = 1$, $p = .51$). See Table 1.

Symptom Analysis

Individuals in the OT group reported significantly more frequent and severe neuromusculoskeletal and movement function symptoms involving difficulties speaking and swallowing ($p = .02$) and hand tremor ($p = .03$) compared to individuals in the No OT group. Individuals with MS in the OT group complained of more severe weakness of the left leg ($p = .04$), but not of the right leg ($p = .24$) than participants in the No OT group. There were no statistically significant differences between the

TABLE 1. Comparison of OT Group and No OT Group Participant Demographics

Participant Demographics	OT n = 12	No OT n = 28	p
Age	47.8 (17.6)*	46.6 (10.6)*	.78
Years of Education	14.9 (10.6)*	13.5 (3.0)*	.18
Gender			
Female (N)	11	20	.16
Male (N)	1	8	
Socioeconomic Status			
Lower (N)	3	12	.51
Middle (N)	6	12	
Upper (N)	3	4	
Ethnicity			
African American (N)	3	11	.38
European American (N)	9	17	
Place of Residence			
Rural (N)	2	11	.16
Suburban (N)	10	17	

*Mean (SD)

OT and No OT groups with regard to the severity of upper extremity weakness, clumsiness of the arms, difficulties walking, or fatigue. These results were confirmed using Fisher LSD procedures. Mean rank MS subject symptom ratings for musculoskeletal and movement-related functions are given in Table 2.

With regard to sensory functions and pain complaints, there were no statistically significant differences between individuals with MS seen for OT services as compared to individuals who were not seen for OT. Specifically, there were no significant differences between groups with regard to reports of double vision, visual acuity, or alterations of sensation involving pain, temperature, touch, paresthesias, or problems with balance. Results concerning participant identification of problems with sensory functions and pain may be found in Table 2. In a similar vein, there were no statistically significant differences between OT group and No OT group with regard to genitourinary or reproductive functions involving bowel and bladder control or sexual dysfunction. The OT group did show a trend to have more frequent reports of uncontrolled urinary urgency than the No OT group ($p = .05$). Results con-

TABLE 2. Mean Rank of Severity and Probability Levels for the OT and No OT Groups for Symptoms Corresponding to Client Factors of Neuromusculoskeletal and Movement-Related Functions, Sensory Functions and Pain

TYPE OF SYMPTOM	OT GROUP Mean Rank	NO OT GROUP Mean Rank	Mann-Whitney U	Corrected Z-score	p
Neuromusculoskeletal and Movement-Related Functions					
Weakness of right arm	22.81	19.39	145.5	−.92	.36
Weakness of left arm	21.69	19.93	160	−.47	.63
Weakness of right leg	23.54	19.04	136	−1.18	.24
Weakness of left leg	25.29	17.64	98.5	−2.04	.04*
Leg stiffness or difficulties walking	23.46	18.46	120.5	−1.32	.19
Tremor	25.58	17.51	95	−2.15	.03*
Clumsiness of arms	22.21	17.46	111.5	−1.31	.19
Difficulty speaking or swallowing	26.04	17.31	89.5	−2.39	.02*
Fatigue	22.21	19.02	135.5	−.84	.39
Sensory Functions and Pain					
Problems with balance	24.27	17.87	113.5	−1.73	.08
Double vision	21.16	18.73	136	−.76	.45
Difficulty in feeling touch	19.83	20.07	160	−.06	.94
Difficulty in feeling heat	20.45	19.80	156.5	−.21	.83
Difficulty in feeling pain	22.50	18.90	132	−.91	.36
Pain/burning sensation anywhere	17.00	21.33	126	−1.10	.27
Unusual/ bizarre sensations	16.72	19.10	105.5	−.61	.55
Visual problem–right eye	20.23	19.20	140.5	−.27	.79
Visual problem–left eye	19.59	19.46	147.5	−.03	.97

* statistically significant at p < .05

cerning other genitourinary or reproductive functions are given in Table 3. There were no statistically significant differences between groups with regard to reports of cognitive and affective problems (see Table 3).

Functional Implications

Of the 40 multiple sclerosis participants, 31 (78%) indicated difficulty with at least one area of occupation (AOC) including activities of

TABLE 3. Mean Rank of Severity and Probability Levels for OT and No OT Groups for Symptoms Corresponding to Client Factors of Mental, Genitourinary and Reproductive Functions

TYPE OF SYMPTOM	OT GROUP Mean Rank	NO OT GROUP Mean Rank	Mann-Whitney U	Corrected Z-score	p
Genitourinary and Reproductive Functions					
Uncontrolled urinary urgency	25.13	17.72	100.5	1.94	.05
Incomplete bladder emptying	24.21	17.33	99.5	−1.88	.06
Constipation	22.15	18.28	124.5	−1.03	.30
Loss of bladder control	21.13	18.09	119.5	−.86	.43
Loss of bowel control	19.67	20.15	158	−.14	.88
Sexual dysfunction	22.87	19.48	139.5	−.87	.38
Mental Functions (Affective, Cognitive and Perceptual)					
Difficulty with memory	23.04	19.28	142.5	−.95	.34
Difficulty with calculation	23.33	16.92	98	−1.79	.07
Difficulty reasoning or thinking	22.29	18.21	122.5	−1.11	.27
Symptoms of depression	19.5	19.5	156	0	.99

* statistically significant at p < .05

daily living, instrumental activities of daily living and work. The most frequently identified AOC, from most to least frequent included functional mobility, work, community mobility, meal preparation and cleanup, dressing, talking, bathing and grooming. Although a greater percentage of the OT group reported functional problems, there was no significant difference between groups with regard to the proportion of individuals who had some problem with AOC ($p > .05$). Within the OT group, only two individuals (2/12 or 17%) reported no functional problems while seven of the 28 (25%) in the No OT group reported no functional problems.

When data were analyzed using group means combined across all functional categories, significantly more MS subjects in the OT group reported functional impairments across all seven categories of activities of daily living (ADL) than MS subjects not receiving OT services: OT group = 46.14% (mean proportion of subjects across all seven ADL categories) vs. No OT group = 28% (mean proportion of subjects across all seven ADL categories) (Chi-square = 6.95, $df = 1$, $p = .008$). "Other" and "No Problems Identified" were not included in this analysis. Individuals in the OT group reported more frequent functional impairments than those in the No OT group in every ADL category including difficulties in walking, working, cooking, driving, dressing, swallowing/speaking, and bathing/grooming. Although more individuals in the OT group complained of difficulties in getting dressed (30%) than in the No OT group (24%), this difference did not reach statistical significance ($p = .71$). The percentage of MS subjects who reported problems with AOCs, Chi-square results, and associated p-values are given for the seven functional impairment areas, as well as for the "Other" and "No Problems Identified" categories, in Table 4.

Participants also reported (wrote in) difficulties in performing functional activities other than the choice of responses in the questionnaire. These were classified as "Other" functional problems. The OT group reported difficulties cleaning the house, shopping, and handwriting. The No OT group reported problems in housekeeping, jogging, and performing yard work.

DISCUSSION

Individuals with multiple sclerosis (MS) who were referred to and participated in occupational therapy (OT) reported more severe neuromusculoskeletal and movement-related problems than individuals with MS who did not receive OT services. There were no significant differences between groups in self-rated symptom severity involving sensory functions, pain, cognition, or mood. Thus, our hypothesis that individuals who were referred to and received OT services would complain of more severe symptoms of MS than individuals who were not seen for OT was not supported. Although individuals who were referred to and received OT services tended to have more severe symptom ratings across all four symptom categories relative to individuals who were not seen by OT, these differences in symptom severity ratings did not reach statistical significance for three of the four symptom categories (refer to Tables 2 and 3).

However, hypothesis 2 (that there would be differences in the symptoms between individuals referred and not referred to OT) was supported. Individuals with MS who were referred to and received OT services reported more severe musculoskeletal and movement-related problems and less severe difficulties in the areas of sensory functions, pain, cog-

TABLE 4. Frequency Reported for Functional Difficulties and Corresponding Areas of Occupation for Participants with Multiple Sclerosis in the OT and No OT Groups

Functional Difficulties	Corresponding Areas of Occupation	OT Group	No OT Group	Chi-Square	p
Walking	Functional Mobility	7/10 (70%)	10/21 (48%)	10.00	.002*
Working	Work	7/10 (70%)	10/21 (48%)	10.00	.002*
Cooking	Meal Preparation & Cleanup	5/10 (50%)	6/21 (29%)	9.23	.002*
Driving	Community Mobility	6/10 (60%)	6/21 (29%)	19.45	.0001*
Dressing	Dressing	3/10 (30%)	5/21 (24%)	0.14	.71
Talking	Information Exchange+	2/10 (20%)	2/21 (9%)	4.88	.03*
Bathing/ Grooming	Bathing/ Grooming	2/10 (20%)	2/21 (9%)	4.88	.03*
Other	Other Functional Problems	3/10 (30%)	8/21 (38%)	4.88	.03*
No Problems Identified		2/12 (17%)	7/28 (25%)	0.33	.56

*statistically significant at p < .05
+In the OT Practice Framework: Domain and Process, information exchange is considered a performance skill rather than an area of occupation.

nition, or affective problems. These symptoms clearly distinguished the OT group from the No OT group. While the more severe problems identified by the OT group (tremor, weakness in left leg and difficulty speaking or swallowing) reflected some of the physical skills necessary to be safe and successful in areas of occupation, other symptoms that influence function (balance, weakness and clumsiness of the arms, fatigue, memory, reasoning or thinking, and calculations) and are amenable to occupational therapy were not identified as discriminators between the two groups. Fatigue was rated among the highest severity levels compared with other symptoms for both the OT and No OT groups. However, there was no significant difference in the number of individuals referred to occupational therapy for fatigue even though there is evidence in the literature that indicates OT intervention may be beneficial for this problem (Mathiowetz et al., 2001).

Of the 31 multiple sclerosis (MS) participants who indicated some difficulty with areas of occupation at the time they responded to the questionnaire, 12 (30%) reported seeing an occupational therapist. This percentage is higher than previous studies for persons with MS (Fawcett et al., 1994; Freeman & Thompson, 2000) and may be attributed to the participants being from a clinical situation in which OT was readily accessible. The most frequent difficulties identified by participants were in the areas of IADLs. Individuals who reported having difficulty in walking, working, cooking, driving, talking, bathing, and grooming were seen for OT at a greater frequency than those who were not seen for OT. Thus the last hypothesis, that more individuals with MS who were referred to and seen for OT would report more difficulties across multiple functional areas than individuals not seen for OT was supported by these results. This is consistent with one of the findings by Finlayson and DalMonte (2002) who found the more functional limitations an individual with MS had the more likely the individual was to participate in OT. It is important to note, however, in the present study no significant differences were found with regard to participation in OT based upon difficulties with dressing, which is a primary area of intervention for occupational therapy.

Implications for Occupational Therapy Practice and Research

In the current study a significant proportion of those who participated in occupational therapy had difficulty in working, walking, driving, and cooking. Practitioners working within MS clinics may be better prepared to meet the needs of individuals with MS by ensuring that evaluations and interventions adequately address these areas of occupation. Occupational therapy practitioners typically employ therapeutic interventions to enhance functional independence in areas of occupation (Youngstrom et al., 2002). For example, Dyck and Jongbloed (2000) suggest the ability to work can be enhanced by modifying the work environment, educating employers, and by using other energy saving techniques in women with MS who are already employed. Vocational rehabilitation interventions outlined by Fraser, Clemmons and Bennett (2002) address sensory, motor, and cognitive impairments that negatively influence success in the workplace and are similar to those services provided by OT practitioners. OT services also include addressing the underlying problems that influence functional independence. Copperman, Forwell and Hugos (2002) identified typical symptoms addressed in OT with suggested treatment for enhancing function for individuals with

MS related to fatigue, weakness, cognition problems, pain, spasticity, and adjustment to the disease.

In this investigation, there were no significant differences between the OT and No OT groups with regard to impairments in sensory function, pain, cognition, or mood; these client factors are, however, within the scope of occupational therapy practice. This finding may be due to a variety of factors such as the limited sample size, participant concerns about cost and reimbursement, or a lack of awareness on the part of referral sources regarding the scope of services and OT interventions for individuals with MS.

Limitations

This study included a small convenient sample of people with MS who had attended an MS clinic, and thus, cannot be generalized to larger populations with absolute confidence. In addition, no comment can be made on the individuals who did not respond, and no information is available on the extent to which they are similar to or different from the respondents.

While this study looked at individuals who were referred to and were seen by OT versus those who were not seen by OT, it is important to note that some individuals may have been referred to OT but have had obstacles such as access, transportation, or reimbursement that could have prevented participation in services after referral. Other factors, such as time since diagnosis, may have influenced the likelihood of referral to OT and should be investigated in future studies. Individuals who have had MS for longer periods of time or more hospitalizations may have acquired more problems and may be more likely to access more diverse health services such as OT. Future studies should investigate these factors.

CONCLUSION

This study compared the signs, symptoms and functional impairments of subjects with MS who were seen in a MS Clinic and who participated in occupational therapy to those who did not participate in OT. In this study, individuals with more severe musculoskeletal and movement-related symptoms and those who reported difficulties across multiple functional areas were most likely to be seen by OT. There was no significant difference in the referral and use of OT by individuals with MS who reported difficulties in areas commonly addressed by OT such as dressing, fatigue, balance and cognition. While OT has been of benefit to individuals with MS, additional research that includes analysis of actual functional outcomes for individuals seen by OT for difficulties in areas of occupation and underlying client factors that influence safety, independence, efficiency and quality of life is warranted.

REFERENCES

Amato, M. P., Ponziani, G., Pracucci, G., Bracco, L., Siracusa, G., & Amaducci, L. (1995). Cognitive impairment in early-onset multiple sclerosis: Pattern, predictors, and impact on everyday life in a 4-year follow-up. *Archives of Neurology*, 52, (2), 168-172.

Baker, N. A. & Tickle-Degnen, L. (2001). The effectiveness of physical, psychological, and functional interventions in treating clients with multiple sclerosis: A meta-analysis. *American Journal of Occupational Therapy*, 55, (3), 324-31.

Copperman, L. F., Forwell, S. J., & Hugos, L. (2002). Neurodegenerative diseases. In C. A. Trombley & M. V. Radomski (Eds.) *Occupational Therapy for Physical Dysfunction* (5th ed. pp 885-96). Philadelphia: Lippincott Williams & Wilkins.

Dyck, I. & Jongbloed, L. (2000). Women with multiple sclerosis and employment issues: A focus on social and institutional environments. *Canadian Journal of Occupational Therapy*, 67, (5), 337-46.

Fawcett, J., Sidney, J. S., Hanson, M. J. S., & Riley-Lawless, K. (1994). Use of alternative health therapies by people with multiple sclerosis: An exploratory study. *Holistic Nurse Practice*, 8, (2), 36-42.

Finlayson, M. & DalMonte, J. (2002). Predicting the use of occupational therapy services among people with multiple sclerosis in Atlantic Canada. *Canadian Journal of Occupational Therapy*, 69, (4), 239-48.

Finlayson, M., Guglielmello, L., & Liefer, K. (2001). Describing and predicting the possession of assistive devices among persons with multiple sclerosis. *American Journal of Occupational Therapy*, 55, (5), 545-51.

Freeman, J. A., Langdon, D. W., Hobart, J. C., & Thompson, A. J. (1997). The impact of inpatient rehabilitation on progressive multiple sclerosis. *Annals of Neurology*, 42, (2), 236-44.

Freeman, J. A. & Thompson, A. J. (2000). Community services in multiple sclerosis: Still a matter of chance. *Journal of Neurology, Neurosurgery, & Psychiatry*, 69, (6), 728-32.

Fraser, R. T., Clemmons, D. C., & Bennett, F. (2002). Multiple sclerosis: Psychosocial and vocational interventions. New York: Demos Medical Publishing.

Gillen, G. (2002). Case report: Improving mobility and community access in an adult with ataxia. *American Journal of Occupational Therapy*, 56, (4), 462-66.

Glazier, R. H., Dalby, D. M., Badley, E. M., Hawker, G. A., Bell, M. J., Buchbinder, R., & Lineker, S. C. (1996). Management of the early and late presentations of rheumatoid arthritis: A survey of Ontario primary care physicians. *Canadian Medical Association Journal*, 155, (6), 679-87.

Gulick, E. E. (1998). Symptom and activities of daily living trajectory in multiple sclerosis: A 10-year study. *Nursing Research, 47*, (3), 137-146.

Hollingshead, A.B. (1957). *Two-factor Index of Social Position*. New Haven, CT: Yale Station.

Lou, J., Classen, S., & Peirce, C. (2002). Wellness and rehabilitation programs for people living with multiple sclerosis. *Multiple Sclerosis Foundation Focus, 4*, (2), 5-7.

Mathiowetz, V., Matuska, K., & Murphy, M. E. (2001). Efficacy of an energy conservation course for persons with multiple sclerosis. *Archives of Physical Medicine Rehabilitation, 82*, 449-56.

Paty, D. W. & Ebers, G. C. (1998). *Multiple Sclerosis*. Philadelphia: F. A. Davis.

Soderback, I. & Paulsson, E. H. (1997). A needs assessment for referral to occupational therapy: Nurses' judgment in acute cancer care. *Cancer Nursing: An International Journal for Cancer Care, 20* (4), 267-73.

Somerset, M., Sharp, D., & Campbell, R. (2002). Multiple sclerosis and quality of life: A qualitative investigation. *Journal of Health Services & Research Policy, 7* (3), 151-159.

van den Noort, S. & Holland, N. J. (1999). *Multiple Sclerosis in Clinical Practice*. New York: Demos Medical Publishing.

Youngstrom, M.J., Brayman, S.J., Anthony, P., Brinson, M., Brownrigg, S., Clark, G.F., Roley, S.S., Sellers, J., Van Slyke, N.L., Desmarais, S.M., Oldham, J., Radomski, M.V., Hertfelder, S.D. (2002, Nov.-Dec.) Occupational therapy practice framework: Domain and process. [Journal Article. Bibliography. Glossary. Standards. Tables/Charts.] *American Journal of Occupational Therapy.* 56(6) : 609-39.

Self-Report Assessment
of Fatigue in Multiple Sclerosis:
A Critical Evaluation

Daphne Kos, MSc
Eric Kerckhofs, PhD
Pierre Ketelaer, MD
Marijke Duportail, OT
Guy Nagels, MD
Marie D'Hooghe, MD
Godelieve Nuyens, PhD

SUMMARY. Fatigue is among the most common and disabling symptoms of multiple sclerosis. Clinicians usually assess fatigue by asking

Daphne Kos is Master in Occupational Therapy, Vrije Universiteit Brussel, Department Physical Therapy, Rehabilitation Research, Laarbeeklaan 103, B-1090 Brussels, Belgium (E-mail: Daphne.Kos@vub.ac.be) and also affiliated with the National Multiple Sclerosis Centre, Vanheylenstraat 16, B-1820 Melsbroek, Belgium (E-mail: d.kos@pandora.be). Eric Kerckhofs is affiliated with Vrije Universiteit Brussel, Department Physical Therapy, Rehabilitation Research, Brussels, Belgium (E-mail: ekerckh@vub.ac.be).

Pierre Ketelaer (E-mail: p.ketelaer@ms-centrum.be), Marijke Duportail (E-mail: marijke.duportail@pandora.be), Guy Nagels (E-mail: gnagels@uia.ua.ac.be), Marie D'Hooghe (E-mail: mb.dhooghe@ms-centrum.be), and Godelieve Nuyens (E-mail: lieve.nuyens@flok.kuleuven.ac.be) are all affiliated with the National Multiple Sclerosis Centre, Vanheylenstraat 16, B-1820 Melsbroek, Belgium.

The authors wish to thank Marcia Finlayson, PhD, for the helpful comments on earlier versions of the manuscript.

This work was supported by a PhD grant from the organisation Wetenschappelijk Onderzoek in Multiple Sclerose (WOMS).

[Haworth co-indexing entry note]: "Self-Report Assessment of Fatigue in Multiple Sclerosis: A Critical Evaluation." Kos, Daphne et al. Co-published simultaneously in *Occupational Therapy in Health Care* (The Haworth Press, Inc.) Vol. 17, No. 3/4, 2003, pp. 45-62; and: *Occupational Therapy Practice and Research with Persons with Multiple Sclerosis* (ed: Marcia Finlayson) The Haworth Press, Inc., 2003, pp. 45-62. Single or multiple copies of this article are available for a fee from The Haworth Document Delivery Service [1-800-HAWORTH, 9:00 a.m. - 5:00 p.m. (EST). E-mail address: docdelivery@haworthpress.com].

10.1300/J003v17n03_04

people to describe and rate their fatigue in a self-report instrument. This paper evaluates the clinical usefulness and the scientific properties of a selection of various self-report instruments for fatigue. To be selected, instruments had to assess fatigue or a related concept, have some published information on reliability and validity, be used in at least one clinical trial of fatigue with people with multiple sclerosis, and demonstrate validity in people with MS. Five fatigue specific scales and four subscales of quality of life instruments were selected and evaluated. In occupational therapy, the fatigue subscales or items of quality of life measurements give limited information about the quality of fatigue. The selection of an instrument may depend on the clinical setting or trial design. *[Article copies available for a fee from The Haworth Document Delivery Service: 1-800-HAWORTH. E-mail address: <docdelivery@haworthpress.com> Website: <http://www.HaworthPress.com> © 2003 by The Haworth Press, Inc. All rights reserved.]*

KEYWORDS. Fatigue, assessment, self-report, multiple sclerosis

INTRODUCTION

Fatigue is reported as the most common and disabling symptom of multiple sclerosis (Bergamaschi, Romani, Versino, Poli, & Cosi, 1997; Freal, Kraft, & Coryell, 1984; Multiple Sclerosis Society, 1997; National Multiple Sclerosis Society, 1997). It has a major impact on work, social and family life, as well as on overall quality of life (Fisk, Pontefract, Ritvo, Archibald, & Murray, 1994; Iriarte, Katsamakis, & de Castro, 1999; Provinciali, Ceravolo, Bartolini, Logullo, & Danni, 1999; Jackson, Quaal, & Reeves, 1991).

MS-related fatigue comes on easily, worsens with heat, interferes with physical functioning and role performance, and is present at all stages of disease (Krupp, Alvarez, LaRocca, & Scheinberg, 1998). A panel of MS researchers and clinicians defined fatigue as "a subjective lack of physical and/or mental energy that is perceived by the individual or caregiver to interfere with usual and desired activities" (Multiple Sclerosis Council for Clinical Practice Guidelines, 1998, p. 2). This description implies that fatigue is a subjective symptom and impairs the ability to participate in self-care, work or leisure activities. This places fatigue in the domain of occupational therapists, who are educated to minimize the interference of impairments with daily life.

Despite more than 15 years of investigation, no definite mechanism underlying the MS-related fatigue has been found. Possible management strategies include (a combination of) medication, "energy management," cooling, exercise, coping and behavioral modification (Branas, Jordan, Fry-Smith, Burls, & Hyde, 2000; Schwid, Covington, Segal, & Goodman, 2002). Before starting a tailor-made intervention, an evaluation of fatigue should be carried out thoroughly.

The Evaluation of Fatigue

Although it is complicated because of the subjectivity and multidimensionality of the symptom (Flachenecker et al., 2002), fatigue can be assessed by either self-report or performance-based measures. Self-report instruments request people to describe and rate their fatigue, while the sustained level of physical or mental performance observed over time is assessed in performance based measures (Chan, 1999; Elkins, Krupp, & Scherl, 2000; Krupp & Elkins, 2000).

The measurement of fatigue on the basis of performance can be valuable for both clinical and research purposes. In occupational therapy practice, however, the assessment of fatigue-related performance is time consuming, costly, and often unrealistic. Though such measures offer important corroborating data unbiased by self-reported perceptions of fatigue, a review of such instruments is beyond the scope of this article.

Different self-report fatigue assessment tools have been developed during the past decade. Most of them are fatigue-specific; others are part of quality of life instruments. In addition to the fatigue-specific assessment, it is crucial to evaluate other symptoms that may contribute to fatigue, such as mood, pain, poor sleep or side-effects of medication (Krupp & Elkins, 2000).

To select an appropriate assessment tool, both clinical usefulness and scientific soundness should be considered (Table 1). This article reviews the clinical and scientific properties of the existing self-report measures for fatigue, applicable in individuals with multiple sclerosis. Using well-evaluated instruments is crucial to evidence-based practice. Assessing the impact of occupational therapy intervention–like teaching energy management strategies–requires an appropriate fatigue assessment tool. Moreover, the choice of an outcome measure determines to a large extent the effectiveness of the treatment (Hobart, Lamping, & Thompson, 1996).

TABLE 1. Evaluation of a Clinical Outcome Measure for Fatigue

Criterion	Description
Clinical usefulness	
Availability	The instrument should be available for use in daily practice.
Ease of administration	The test should be easy and quick to administer.
Scientific properties	
Level of measurement	The score should be quantitative and the distance between points on the scale should be known (interval scale).
Applicability to patients with variation in the symptom	The instrument should avoid ceiling and floor effects.
Reliability	The self-report measure should be internally consistent and stable over time.
Validity	The instrument should measure what it intends to measure (fatigue – impact of fatigue on daily functioning etc.).
Responsiveness	The instrument should be able to detect clinically significant change.

Sources: (Fischer et al., 1999; Hobart et al., 1996; Whitaker et al., 1995; Rudick et al., 1996)

METHOD

An electronic search of the literature in PubMed, scanning data to November 2002, provided our selection of fatigue assessment tools, which was based on four criteria: Instruments had to assess fatigue or a related concept, have some published information on reliability and validity, demonstrate validity in people with MS, and be used in at least one clinical trial of fatigue with people with multiple sclerosis.

RESULTS

Selected Instruments

Table 2 shows the eighteen detected instruments that met at least one of the selection criteria. The fatigue specific scales and health status measures are separately ordered from most to least frequent use. Scales that met all criteria are marked in italics and therefore were included for further evaluation.

1. The Fatigue Severity Scale (FSS) (Krupp, LaRocca, Muir-Nash, & Steinberg, 1989)–a questionnaire which asks people to rate their agreement with nine statements–is the most commonly used measure for fatigue in multiple sclerosis. The FSS evaluates the severity, frequency and impact of fatigue on daily life.
2. The 40-item Fatigue Impact Scale (FIS) (Fisk, Pontefract et al., 1994) measures, in three subscales, the impact of fatigue on physical, cognitive and psychosocial functioning.
3. The Modified Fatigue Impact Scale (MFIS) (Multiple Sclerosis Council for Clinical Practice Guidelines, 1998) is derived from the FIS, and consists of 21 items. This scale is a component of the Multiple Sclerosis Quality of Life Inventory and, like the FIS, evaluates the impact of fatigue on physical, cognitive and psychosocial functioning.
4. The Fatigue Descriptive Scale (FDS) (Iriarte et al., 1999) is a five-item instrument to evaluate the severity, frequency and quality of fatigue. The influence of heat on fatigue (the so-called Uhthoff phenomenon) and the spontaneity of fatigue complaints are also considered.
5. The 29-item Fatigue Assessment Instrument (FAI) (Schwartz, Jandorf, & Krupp, 1993) (in other publications mentioned as Mul-

tiple Sclerosis Specific-Fatigue Scale, MSS-FS) is composed of eight of the nine items of the FSS and addresses quantitative and qualitative components of fatigue, in four subscales.

6. The Short Form-36 (SF-36) (Ware, Jr. & Sherbourne, 1992; McHorney, Ware, Jr., & Raczek, 1993) is acknowledged as the gold standard generic health status measure, with an "energy and vitality" dimension.

7. The Guy's Neurological Disability Scale (GNDS) (Sharrack & Hughes, 1999) is a disability measure developed for use in multiple sclerosis; it consists of 12 categories, including fatigue.

8. The Illness Intrusiveness Ratings Scale (IIRS) (Devins et al., 1983) asks people to rate the interference of the illness with their life, covering the domains of relationships and personal development, intimacy and instrumental (e.g., work, active recreation).

9. The 59-item quality of life instrument for use with people with MS, the Functional Assessment of Multiple Sclerosis (FAMS) (Cella et al., 1996), is divided into 6 subscales, including thinking/fatigue.

Evaluation of Selected Instruments

The evaluation of the selected instruments is based on the clinical and scientific criteria as stated in Table 1. The clinical usefulness is determined by availability and ease of administration, which influences the cost-effectiveness of the instrument.

Evaluation of scientific properties addresses level of measurement, applicability to people with a variation in fatigue, reliability, validity and responsiveness (Fischer et al., 1999; Hobart et al., 1996; Whitaker, McFarland, Rudge, & Reingold, 1995; Rudick et al., 1996).

Clinical usefulness. All scales are available in literature, most of them in different languages, like FSS, FIS, FDS, FAI, SF-36 and FAMS. All scales can be filled out and scored in 10-45 minutes. The tools are rather brief (Table 3), except for the Fatigue Impact Scale, which consists of 40 items and therefore could provoke fatigue. The shorter (21-item) version–Modified Fatigue Impact Scale–may be more appropriate for this criterion. Other scales have fewer items, varying from 4 to 29 items.

A higher total score means a person is more fatigued, except for the vitality subscale of SF-36 with a higher score implying more vitality, thus less fatigue. Whereas the total score is usually the sum of all items, the Fatigue Descriptive Scale has a more complex way of rating. The spontaneity of a fatigue complaint has a great impact on the total score

TABLE 2. Instruments Assessing Fatigue; Those Included for Further Evaluation Are Marked in Italics. (V: validated for people with MS; CT: clinical trial concerning fatigue in multiple sclerosis; #CT: number of clinical trials in multiple sclerosis)

Scale	V	CT	# CT
Fatigue specific scales			
Fatigue Severity Scale (FSS) (Krupp et al., 1989)	+	+	22
Fatigue Impact Scale (FIS) (Fisk, Pontefract et al., 1994)	+	+	11
Modified Fatigue Impact Scale (MFIS) (Multiple Sclerosis Council for Clinical Practice Guidelines, 1998)	+	+	3
Visual Analogue Scale for Fatigue (VAS-F) (Lee, Hicks, & Nino-Murcia, 1991)	–	+	2
Fatigue Descriptive Scale (FDS) (Iriarte & de Castro, 1994)	+	+	2
Fatigue Assessment Instrument (FAI) = Multiple Sclerosis Specific Fatigue Scale (MSS-FS) (Schwartz et al., 1993)	+	+	2
Fatigue Rating Scale (FRS) (Chalder et al., 1993)	–	+	2
Multidimensional Assessment of Fatigue (MAF) (Belza, Henke, Yelin, Epstein, & Gilliss, 1993)	–	+	1
Epworth Sleepiness Scale (ESS) (Johns, 1991)	–	+	1
Piper Self-report Fatigue Scale (PFS) (Piper et al., 1989)	–	–	0
Fatigue Energy Consciousness Energized and Sleepiness (FACES) (Shapiro et al., 2002)	–	–	0
Health status measures			
Short Form-36 (SF-36) (Ware & Sherbourne, 1992)	+	+	4
Guy's Neurological Disability Scale (GNDS) (Sharrack & Hughes, 1999)	+	+	3
Sickness Impact Profile (SIP) (Bergner et al., 1976; Pollard et al., 1976)	–*	+	2
Profile of Mood States (POMS) (McNair, Lorr, & Droppleman, 1971)	–	+	1
Illness Intrusiveness Ratings Scale (IIRS) (Devins et al., 1983)	+	+	1
Functional Assessment of Multiple Sclerosis (FAMS) (Cella et al., 1996)	+	+	1
Checklist of Individual Strength (CIS) (Vercoulen et al., 1994)	–	–	0

* Sample with rehabilitation medicine patients and outpatients with chronic problems; the disease is not described

51

TABLE 3. Number of Items, Score Range, Maximum Total Score, Scoring Direction and Dimensions of Fatigue Assessment Tools

Scale	# of items	Score range	Maximum total score	Scoring direction	Dimensions
Fatigue Severity Scale	9	1-7 (Likert)	63	↑	Modality, severity, frequency, impact on daily life
Fatigue Impact Scale	40	0-4 (Likert)	160	↑	Cognitive, psychosocial, physical impact
Modified Fatigue Impact Scale	21	0-4 (Likert)	84	↑	Cognitive, psychosocial, physical impact
Fatigue Descriptive Scale	5	0-3	17	↑	Modality, spontaneity, severity, frequency and Uhthoff phenomenon*
Fatigue Assessment Instrument = Multiple Sclerosis Specific-Fatigue Scale	29	1-7 (Likert)	203	↑	Fatigue severity, situation, consequences, responsiveness to rest/sleep
Short Form-36, vitality scale	4	1-6 (Likert)	24	→	Frequency of vitality
Guy's Neurological Disability Scale, fatigue subscale	5	0-1	5	↑	Frequency, impact on daily activities
Illness Intrusiveness Ratings Scale	13	1-7 (Likert)	91	↑	Interference of illness with 13 domains of life
Functional Assessment of Multiple Sclerosis, subscale thinking/fatigue	9 (5 fatigue items)	0-4 (Likert)	36 (fatigue items only: 20)	↑	Modality, consequences

* Uhthoff phenomenon: the influence of temperature on symptoms.
↑ or ↓: scoring direction indicating increased (impact of) fatigue

in the FDS, and implies an interview is necessary for this scale. This could influence the cost-effectiveness of the scale.

Scientific properties. Level of measurement: The level of measurement is mainly ordinal (Table 3). Except for the Fatigue Descriptive Scale and the Guy's Neurological Disability Scale, all instruments use a Likert scale, as responses are constructed on an agree-disagree continuum. The data from these instruments can be analyzed as if they were interval unless the distribution of scores is severely skewed (Streiner & Norman, 1989). This distribution is usually not described in literature; therefore it is not always possible to evaluate the appropriateness of statistical analyses. Only the SF-36 study reported the distribution, which is normal for the vitality dimension (Freeman, Hobart, Langdon, & Thompson, 2000). The analysis of results with parametric techniques is therefore appropriate.

Applicability to people with a variation in fatigue: The fatigue scales assess various dimensions of fatigue like modality, severity, frequency and impact on daily functioning (Table 3). The original and modified Fatigue Impact Scale only assesses the impact of fatigue on various domains of daily life.

People with multiple sclerosis can vary in the severity, modality or impact of fatigue. A fatigue questionnaire should be able to assess the whole scope of fatigue, which can be evaluated by examining the distribution of results. A ceiling or floor effect exists when responses are severely skewed to the upper or lower end of the scale, respectively. This implies it is hard to measure an improvement, a decrease, or a distinction among various high or low scores.

Only one study reported the score distributions of a scale. The vitality and energy subscores of the Short Form-36 (SF-36), showed no marked floor or ceiling effects in multiple sclerosis (Freeman et al., 2000). Though not established here, a floor effect is imaginable when used in the more severely disabled individuals with MS. This also applies to other instruments that assess fatigue impact, as the interference of fatigue with physical functioning is difficult to evaluate when physical abilities are severely limited. This indicates that not only the heterogeneity of fatigue, but also the heterogeneity of the MS population, in terms of severity and clinical course (Wingerchuk & Weinshenker, 2000), influence the use of assessment tools.

Reliability: A reliable self-report measure is internally consistent and stable over time. The internal consistency is the extent to which items of a scale measure the same concept (Hobart et al., 1996). This is especially important when a total score is calculated by summing all subscores, which is usual for most fatigue scales. If subitems measure different attributes, it does not make sense to interpret them in one total score. But, on the other hand, if items highly correlate with each other, they probably provide the same information, which makes one of them superfluous. Therefore, scale items are considered "homogeneous" if Cronbach's alpha is above .70 but not higher than .90 (Streiner et al., 1989).

Internal consistency was demonstrated in all scales except for the Fatigue Descriptive Scale (Table 4). However, this topic is not relevant in FDS, for this tool is multidimensional and the total score is more complex than a simple summation of the subscores.

Stability over time is measured by test-retest reliability. This is an important topic for self-report measures, because of the possible impulsive response and daily or even hourly fluctuations in fatigue. An instrument should be stable, but sensitive enough to measure changes as well. In the Fatigue Impact Scale (FIS) and Modified Fatigue Impact Scale (MFIS), people are asked to recall the impact of their fatigue during the past four weeks, so fluctuations are not expected, but recall bias is possible. However, no test-retest reliability has been addressed in these scales. Stability over time was rather poor in the Fatigue Assessment Instrument, especially for the subscale "responsiveness to rest/sleep" (r = .29). Fatigue Severity Scale, Short Form-36, Guy's Neurological Disability Scale, Illness Intrusiveness Ratings Scale and Fatigue Assessment of Multiple Sclerosis were all stable measures. For the score of the Fatigue Descriptive Scale is based on an interview, the interrater agreement was applied, which was moderate to good (Kappa = .53 to .81 for various subscales).

Validity: The validity of an instrument is the extent to which it measures the concept it purports to measure, concerning three different types of validity: Content, construct and criterion related validity. As no criterion (Whitaker et al., 1995) is available in fatigue scales, only content and construct validity were evaluated (Hobart et al., 1996).

Content validity is the extent to which an instrument covers the concerned domain and is usually logically judged by an expert (and user) panel. Face validity–a related concept–concerns the extent to which items measure the desired qualities.

All scales, except the Fatigue Descriptive Scale, demonstrated content validity by experts and people with MS. Schwid et al. (2002) argued the limited face validity of the FSS as a fatigue severity measure: Besides the severity, FSS items evaluate the quality and the consequences of fatigue and compare the severity with other MS symptoms without indicating fatigue quality or quantity.

TABLE 4. Comparison of the Scientific Properties of the Fatigue Instruments Selected for Evaluation

Scale	Size of MS sample	Cronbach's alpha	Stability over time	Construct validity	Responsiveness
Fatigue Severity Scale (FSS) (Krupp et al., 1989)	n = 25	.81	r = .84	.47 (VAS)	+
Fatigue Impact Scale (FIS) (Fisk, Pontefract et al., 1994)	n = 105	> .87	NA	.53 (SIP)	NA
(Mathiowetz et al., 2001)	n = 54	NA	NA	NA	+
Modified Fatigue Impact Scale (MFIS) (National Multiple Sclerosis Society, 1997)	n = 300	.81	NA	.47 (SIP)	NA
(Rammohan et al., 2002)	n = 72	NA	NA	NA	+
Fatigue Descriptive Scale (FDS) (Iriarte & de Castro., 1994)	n = 32	NA	K ≥ .53	≥ .66 (FSS)	NA
Fatigue Assessment Instrument (FAI) (Schwartz et al., 1993)	n = 40	≥ .70	r = .29 – .69 (four subscales)	.976 (FSS) −.72 (RIV)	NA
(Krupp et al., 1995)	n = 93	NA	NA	NA	+
Short Form-36 (SF-36) (vitality subscale) (Brazier et al., 1992)	n = 1,643	≥ .85	r > .75	NA	NA
(Freeman et al., 2000)	n = 150	≥ .77	NA	.61 (SF-36, emotional wellbeing) .18 (SF-36, physical functioning)	–
Guy's Neurological Disability Scale (GNDS) (fatigue subscale) (Sharrack & Hughes., 1999)	n = 50	≥ .79	r = .96	NA	+
(Rossier & Ware, 2002)	n = 43	NA	r = .68	.67 (FSS)	NA
Illness Intrusiveness Ratings Scale (IIRS) (Devins et al., 1983)	n = 174	> .65	NA	NA	NA
(Shawaryn et al., 2002)	n = 90	.90	r ≥ .80	.71 (MFIS)	NA
Functional Assessment of Multiple Sclerosis (FAMS), subscale thinking/fatigue (Cella et al., 1996)	n = 377(survey) n = 56 (clinical)	.91	r = .85	−.75 (MDI Veg)	NA

NA: not addressed
VAS: Visual Analogue Scale; SIP: Sickness Impact Profile; RIV: Rand Index of Vitality; MDI
Veg: Multiscale Depression Inventory Vegetative
+: able to detect a statistical significant (p < .01) difference after intervention

55

Construct validation–evidence for measuring the construct it is intented to measure–is mainly achieved by estimating the extent to which the scale correlates with instruments with convergent (similar) or discriminant constructs and by evaluating the ability to distinguish between groups in predictable ways (Hobart et al., 1996). Fatigue scales assess various dimensions of fatigue, as demonstrated by Flachenecker and colleagues (2002), which makes the comparison complex.

Some instruments used FSS to correlate (Table 4), although FSS itself correlated moderately (r = .47 in people with MS, r = 0.50 in healthy persons) with a 100-mm visual analogue scale (VAS) for fatigue severity (Krupp et al., 1989), on which people were asked to indicate the point which best described their fatigue. FSS distinguished fatigue experienced by people with MS from healthy adults (Krupp et al., 1989) and differentiated between fatigued and non-fatigued people with MS (Flachenecker et al., 2002).

Both the Fatigue Impact Scale and Modified Fatigue Impact Scale correlated moderately with Sickness Impact Profile, a 136-item behaviourally based measure of health status (Bergner, Bobbitt, Pollard, Martin, & Gilson, 1976; Pollard, Bobbitt, Bergner, Martin, & Gilson, 1976). FIS was able to differentiate people with MS from controls (Fisk, Ritvo et al., 1994); MFIS was able to distinguish between fatigued and non-fatigued people with MS (Flachenecker et al., 2002).

The Fatigue Descriptive Scale correlated moderately with FSS, although FDS assesses not only fatigue severity. No information about distinction between groups is available (Iriarte et al., 1999; Iriarte & de Castro, 1994).

The Fatigue Assessment Instrument (FAI) is composed of eight of the nine items of the FSS, which explains the high correlation with the latter scale. The fatigue severity subscale of FAI correlated substantially ($-.72$) with the Rand Index of Vitality (RIV). The RIV (Brook et al., 1979) is a subscale of the Rand's Health Insurance Survey that measures energy, with a higher score when people are less fatigued, which explains the negative correlations. The FAI distinguished people with MS from controls and subjects from other diagnostic groups, both in a quantitative and a qualitative way (Schwartz et al., 1993).

As expected, the "energy and vitality" dimension of the Short Form-36 (SF-36) correlated moderately with emotional well-being and poorly with physical function (Freeman et al., 2000) and distinguished between groups with expected health differences (Brazier et al., 1992).

The fatigue subscale of the Guy's Neurological Disability Scale (GNDS) correlated .67 with FSS; divided over a postal and a face-to-face group, the correlation was poor (.40) and good (.84), respectively (Rossier & Wade, 2002).

The Illness Intrusiveness Ratings Scale (IIRS) assesses the interference of the illness with their life in various domains. The good correlation with MFIS demonstrated the related construct (Shawaryn, Schiaffino, LaRocca, & Johnston, 2002).

The thinking/fatigue subscale of the Functional Assessment of Multiple Sclerosis (FAMS) correlated well with the vegetative subscale of the Multiscale Depression Inventory. The authors presumed that people with MS experience an element of depression, which is distinguishable from depressed mood thinking (Cella et al., 1996). As expected, no relationship with neurological dysfunction and social desirability has been found.

Responsiveness: The responsiveness–sensitivity to clinical change– can be determined by measuring the concept at two points in time when clinical changes are expected (Hobart et al., 1996). Across the scales reviewed, the following responsiveness has been documented:

- The Fatigue Severity Scale changed significantly in people receiving fatigue-reducing medication (Krupp et al., 1989).
- FIS indicated a significant change after energy conservation course (Mathiowetz, Matuska, & Murphy, 2001) and with a cooling suit (Flensner & Lindencrona, 2002). MFIS was able to discriminate between treatment with placebo and modafinil (Rammohan et al., 2002) and Prokarin® (Gillson, Richard, Smith, & Wright, 2002).
- The Fatigue Assessment Instrument was able to differentiate between people receiving amantadine and the placebo group (Krupp et al., 1995).
- The overall responsiveness of SF-36 was poor and the vitality subscale showed no significant change after rehabilitation (Freeman et al., 2000).
- The overall responsiveness of Guy's NDS was moderate, although measured in a small sample (n = 15) (Sharrack et al., 1999).

No information about the responsiveness of FDS, IIRS or FAMS was available.

DISCUSSION AND IMPLICATIONS
FOR OCCUPATIONAL THERAPY

Fatigue assessment tools measure different dimensions of fatigue. The choice of an instrument may partly depend on the desired information. While the evaluated instruments provide useful information concerning the nature of fatigue, an occupational therapist is mainly interested in the impact of the symptom on daily living. Therefore the Fatigue Impact Scale and the Modified Fatigue Impact Scale are useful tools, although their stability over time is not established yet. The length of FIS (40 items), however, could provoke fatigue. The MFIS may be a good alternative, but basically has not been retested by Rasch analyses. This could be a topic in future research.

With the obtained information of these scales, an occupational therapist can develop and evaluate tailor-made energy management programs. When interested in the nature of fatigue, scales like Fatigue Severity Scale, Fatigue Descriptive Scale and Fatigue Assessment Instrument can be useful. While FDS requires an interview, FSS and FAI are self-administered. FSS has good scientific properties. FDS is highly correlated with FSS, but no information about the responsiveness of this scale is available. Not all subscales of FAI are stable over time.

The subscales or items of quality of life measurements provide limited information concerning fatigue. Also, these instruments were developed for use as a whole and studied this way; therefore they are less useful in occupational therapy setting. The scales could be valuable as an instrument to detect people with fatigue. The SF-36, GNDS, IIRS and FAMS are reliable and valid instruments, but only GNDS has demonstrated responsiveness, in a small sample.

Although the FACES checklist (Shapiro et al., 2002) is not validated for people with multiple sclerosis yet, the concept is interesting. It is based on the differentiation between fatigue, energy, consciousness, energized and sleepiness (de Rijk, Schreurs, & Bensing, 1999; Iriarte, Subira, & de Castro, 2000; Shapiro et al., 2002; Shapiro, 1998). This distinction is probably one reason why self-report instruments do not correlate well with performance. The different aspects of fatigue and energy being used here are likely to reduce the potential for floor or ceiling effects in the heterogeneous MS population.

CONCLUSION

The assessment of fatigue is difficult, because of its subjectivity and multidimensionality. Self-report instruments assess the subjective experience of frequency, modality, severity of fatigue and the impact on daily life. They also assess dimensions of fatigue in MS, notably physical and mental.

Most of the fatigue specific scales are reliable and valid instruments, but not all of them demonstrate stability and responsiveness. In clinical practice however, where the evolution of a client and the treatment are evaluated, these are crucial topics.

The fatigue subscales or items of quality of life measurements give limited information about the quality of fatigue. These could be useful as a screening instrument.

The selection of an assessment tool may depend on the clinical setting or trial design.

There seems to be a trend to differentiate between various aspects of fatigue like lack of energy, consciousness and sleepiness, but no valid assessment tool for this concept is available for people with multiple sclerosis yet.

To improve the measurement of fatigue, future research should address the fundamental scientific evaluation of the Modified Fatigue Impact Scale and the stability and responsiveness of the (Modified) Fatigue Impact Scale. Also, the clinical usefulness and the scientific properties of the FACES checklist should be evaluated in people with multiple sclerosis.

REFERENCES

Belza, B.L., Henke, C.J., Yelin, E.H., Epstein, W.V., & Gilliss, C.L. (1993). Correlates of fatigue in older adults with rheumatoid arthritis. *Nursing Research, 42 (2)*, 93-99.

Bergamaschi, R., Romani, A., Versino, M., Poli, R., & Cosi, V. (1997). Clinical aspects of fatigue in multiple sclerosis. *Functional Neurology, 12 (5)*, 247-251.

Bergner, M., Bobbitt, R.A., Pollard, W.E., Martin, D.P., & Gilson, B.S. (1976). The sickness impact profile: Validation of a health status measure. *Medical Care, 14 (1)*, 57-67.

Brañas, P., Jordan, R., Fry-Smith, A., Burls, A., & Hyde, C. (2000). Treatments for fatigue in multiple sclerosis: A rapid and systematic review. *Health Technology Assessment, 4 (27)*, 1-61.

Brazier, J.E., Harper, R., Jones, N.M., O' Cathain, A., Thomas, K.J., Usherwood, T. et al. (1992). Validating the SF-36 health survey questionnaire: New outcome measure for primary care. *British Medical Journal, 305*, 160-164.

Brook, R.H., Ware, J.E. Jr., Davies-Avery, A., Stewart, A.L., Donald, C.A., Rogers, W.H. et al. (1979). Overview of adult measures fielded in the Rand's Health Insurance Study. *Medical Care, 17*, (7 suppl) 1-131.

Cella, D.F., Dineen, K., Arnason, B., Reder, A., Webster, K.A., Karabatsos, G. et al. (1996). Validation of the functional assessment of multiple sclerosis, quality of life instrument. *Neurology, 47*, 129-139.

Chalder, T., Berelowitz, G., Pawlikowska, T., Watts, L., Wessely, S., Wright, D. et al. (1993). Development of a fatigue scale. *Journal of Psychosomatic Research, 37 (2)*, 147-153.

Chan, A. (1999). A review of common management strategies for fatigue in multiple sclerosis. *International Journal of Multiple Sclerosis Care*, 2, 13-19.

de Rijk, A.E., Schreurs, K.M., & Bensing, J.M. (1999). What is behind "I'm so tired?" Fatigue experiences and their relations to the quality and quantity of external stimulation. *Journal of Psychosomatic Research*, 47 (6), 509-523.

Devins, G.M., Binik, Y.M., Hutchinson, T.A., Hollomboy, D.J., Barré, P.E., & Guttmann, R.D. (1983). The emotional impact of end-stage renal disease: Importance of patients' perception of intrusiveness and control. *International Journal of Psychiatry in Medicine*, 13, 327-343.

Elkins, L.E., Krupp, L.B., & Scherl, W. (2000). The measurement of fatigue and contributing neuropsychiatric factors. *Seminars in Clinical Neuropsychiatry*, 5 (1), 58-61.

Fischer, J.S., LaRocca, N.G., Miller, D.M., Ritvo, P.G., Andrews, H., & Paty, D. (1999). Recent developments in the assessment of quality of life in multiple sclerosis (MS). *Multiple Sclerosis*, 5 (4), 251-259.

Fisk, J.D., Pontefract, A., Ritvo, P.G., Archibald, C.J., & Murray, T.J. (1994). The impact of fatigue on patients with multiple sclerosis. *Canadian Journal of Neurological Sciences*, 21 (1), 9-14.

Fisk, J.D., Ritvo, P.G., Ross, L., Haase, D.A., Marrie, T.J., & Schlech, W.F. (1994). Measuring the functional impact of fatigue: Initial validation of the fatigue impact scale. *Clinical Infectious Diseases*, 18 (Suppl 1), S79-S83.

Flachenecker, P., Kümpfel, T., Kallmann, B., Gottschalk, M., Grauer, O., Rieckmann, P., Trenkwalder, C., & Toyka, K.V. (2002). Fatigue in multiple sclerosis: A comparison of different rating scales and correlation to clinical parameters. *Multiple Sclerosis*, 8, 523-526.

Flensner, G. & Lindencrona, C. (2002). The cooling-suit: Case studies of its influence on fatigue among eight individuals with multiple sclerosis. *Journal of Advanced Nursing*, 37 (6), 541-550.

Freal, J.E., Kraft, G.H., & Coryell, J.K. (1984). Symptomatic fatigue in multiple sclerosis. *Archives of Physical and Medical Rehabilitation*, 65 (3), 135-138.

Freeman, J.A., Hobart, J.C., Langdon, D.W., & Thompson, A.J. (2000). Clinical appropriateness: A key factor in outcome measure selection: The 36 item short form health survey in multiple sclerosis. *Journal of Neurology, Neurosurgery and Psychiatry*, 68 (2), 150-156.

Gillson, G., Richard, T.L., Smith, R.B., & Wright, J.V. (2002). A double-blind pilot study of the effect of Prokarin on fatigue in multiple sclerosis. *Multiple Sclerosis*, 8 (1), 30-35.

Hobart, J.C., Lamping, D.L., & Thompson, A.J. (1996). Evaluating neurological outcome measures: The bare essentials. *Journal of Neurology, Neurosurgery and Psychiatry*, 60 (2), 127-130.

Iriarte, J. & de Castro, P. (1994). [Proposal of a new scale for assessing fatigue in patients with multiple sclerosis]. *Neurologia*, 9 (3), 96-100.

Iriarte, J., Katsamakis, G., & de Castro, P. (1999). The Fatigue Descriptive Scale (FDS): A useful tool to evaluate fatigue in multiple sclerosis. *Multiple Sclerosis*, 5 (1), 10-16.

Iriarte, J., Subira, M.L., & de Castro, P. (2000). Modalities of fatigue in multiple sclerosis: Correlation with clinical and biological factors. *Multiple Sclerosis*, 6 (2), 124-130.

Jackson, M.F., Quaal, C., & Reeves, M.A. (1991). Effects of multiple sclerosis on occupational and career patterns. *Axone, 13 (1)*, 20-22.

Johns, M.W. (1991). A new method for measuring daytime sleepiness: The Epworth sleepiness scale. *Sleep, 14 (6)*, 540-545.

Krupp, L.B., Alvarez, L.A., LaRocca, N.G., & Scheinberg, L.C. (1988). Fatigue in multiple sclerosis. *Archives of Neurology, 45 (4)*, 435-437.

Krupp, L.B., Coyle, P.K., Doscher, C., Miller, A., Cross, A.H., Jandorf, L. et al. (1995). Fatigue therapy in multiple sclerosis: Results of a double-blind, randomized, parallel trial of amantadine, pemoline, and placebo. *Neurology, 45*, 1956-1961.

Krupp, L.B. & Elkins, L.E. (2000). Fatigue. In J.S. Burks & K.P. Johnson (Eds.). *Multiple Sclerosis: Diagnosis, medical management and rehabilitation* (pp. 291-297) New York: Demos.

Krupp, L.B., LaRocca, N.G., Muir-Nash, J., & Steinberg, A.D. (1989). The fatigue severity scale. Application to patients with multiple sclerosis and systemic lupus erythematosus. *Archives of Neurology, 46 (10)*, 1121-1123.

Lee, K. A., Hicks, G., & Nino-Murcia, G. (1991). Validity and reliability of a scale to assess fatigue. *Psychiatry Research, 36 (3)*, 291-298.

Mathiowetz, V., Matuska, K.M., & Murphy, M.E. (2001). Efficacy of an energy conservation course for persons with multiple sclerosis. *Archives of Physical and Medical Rehabilitation, 82 (4)*, 449-456.

McHorney, C.A., Ware, J.E., Jr., & Raczek, A.E. (1993). The MOS 36-Item Short-Form Health Survey (SF-36): II. Psychometric and clinical tests of validity in measuring physical and mental health constructs. *Medical Care, 31(3)*, 247-263.

McNair, D., Lorr, M., & Droppleman, L. (1971). EDITS Manual for the profile of mood states. San Diego (CA): Educational and industrial testing service.

Multiple Sclerosis Council for Clinical Practice Guidelines (1998). Fatigue and multiple sclerosis: Evidence-based management strategies for fatigue in multiple sclerosis. Washington, DC: Paralyzed Veterans of America.

Multiple Sclerosis Society (1997). *Symptom Management Survey Multiple Sclerosis.* United Kingdom: unpublished report.

National Multiple Sclerosis Society (1997). *Multiple Sclerosis Quality of Life Inventory: Technical Supplement.* Unpublished report, available on request (nicholas. larocca@nmss.org).

Piper, B.F., Lindsey, A.M., Dodd, M.J., Ferketich, S., Paul, S.M., & Weller, S. (1989). The development of an instrument to measure the subjective dimension of fatigue. *Key Aspects of Comfort: Management of Pain, Fatigue, and Nausea* (pp. 199-208). New York: Springer.

Pollard, W.E., Bobbitt, R.A., Bergner, M., Martin, D.P., & Gilson, B.S. (1976). The Sickness Impact Profile: Reliability of a health status measure. *Medical Care, 14 (2)*, 146-155.

Provinciali, L., Ceravolo, M. G., Bartolini, M., Logullo, F., & Danni, M. (1999). A multidimensional assessment of multiple sclerosis: Relationships between disability domains. *Acta Neurologica Scandinavica, 100 (3)*, 156-162.

Rammohan, K.W., Rosenberg, J.H., Lynn, D.J., Blumenfeld, A.M., Pollak, C.P., & Nagaraja, H.N. (2002). Efficacy and safety of modafinil (Provigil) for the treatment of fatigue in multiple sclerosis: A two centre phase 2 study. *Journal of Neurology, Neurosurgery and Psychiatry, 72 (2)*, 179-183.

Rossier, P. & Wade, D.T. (2002). The Guy's Neurological Disability Scale in patients with multiple sclerosis: A clinical evaluation of its reliability and validity. *Clinical Rehabilitation, 16 (1),* 75-95.

Rudick, R., Antel, J., Confavreux, C., Cutter, G., Ellison, G., Fischer, J. et al. (1996). Clinical outcomes assessment in multiple sclerosis. *Annals of Neurology, 40 (3),* 469-479.

Schwartz, J.E., Jandorf, L., & Krupp, L.B. (1993). The measurement of fatigue: A new instrument. *Journal of Psychosomatic Research, 37 (7),* 753-762.

Schwid, S.R., Covington, M., Segal, B.M., & Goodman, A.D. (2002). Fatigue in multiple sclerosis: Current understanding and future directions. *Journal of Rehabilitation Research and Development, 39 (2),* 211-224.

Shapiro, C.M. (1998). Fatigue: How many types and how common? *Journal of Psychosomatic Research, 45,* 1-3.

Shapiro, C.M., Flanigan, M., Fleming, J.A., Morehouse, R., Moscovitch, A., Plamondon, J. et al. (2002). Development of an adjective checklist to measure five FACES of fatigue and sleepiness. Data from a national survey of insomniacs. *Journal of Psychosomatic Research, 52 (6),* 467-473.

Sharrack, B. & Hughes, R.A. (1999). The Guy's Neurological Disability Scale (GNDS): A new disability measure for multiple sclerosis. *Multiple Sclerosis, 5 (4),* 223-233.

Shawaryn, M.A., Schiaffino, K.M., LaRocca, N.G., & Johnston, M.V. (2002). Determinants of health-related quality of life in multiple sclerosis: The role of illness intrusiveness. *Multiple Sclerosis, 8 (4),* 310-318.

Streiner, D.L. & Norman, G.R. (1989). Health measurement scales. New York: Oxford University Press.

Vercoulen, J.H., Swanink, C.M., Fennis, J.F., Galama, J.M., van der Meer, J.W., & Bleijenberg, G. (1994). Dimensional assessment of chronic fatigue syndrome. *Journal of Psychosomatic Research, 38 (3),* 383-392.

Ware, J.E., Jr. & Sherbourne, C.D. (1992). The MOS 36-item short-form health survey (SF-36). I. Conceptual framework and item selection. *Medical Care, 30 (6),* 473-483.

Whitaker, J.N., McFarland, H.F., Rudge, P., & Reingold, S.C. (1995). Outcomes assessment in multiple sclerosis clinical trials: A critical analysis. *Multiple Sclerosis, 1 (1),* 37-47.

Wingerchuk, D.M. & Weinshenker, B.G. (2000). Multiple sclerosis: Epidemiology, genetics, classification, natural history, and clinical outcome measures. *Neuroimaging Clinics of North America, 10 (4),* 611-624.

The Effect of Wheelchair Use
on the Quality of Life of Persons
with Multiple Sclerosis

Rachel Devitt, BHSc, OT Reg (Ont)
Betty Chau, BSc, OT Reg (Ont)
Jeffrey W. Jutai, PhD, CPsych

SUMMARY. This pilot study describes the effect of wheelchair use on the quality of life of persons with multiple sclerosis (MS), and examines the clinical utility of the Psychosocial Impact of Assistive Devices Scale

---

Rachel Devitt is affiliated with the Bridgepoint Health, 14 St. Mathews Road, Toronto, ON, Canada, M4M 2B5 (E-mail: rachel.devitt@utoronto.ca).

Betty Chau is affiliated with the North York General Hospital, 4001 Leslie Street, Toronto, Ontario, Canada, M2K 1E1 (E-mail:chau_betty@hotmail.com).

Jeffrey W. Jutai is Associate Professor, Faculty of Health Sciences, School of Occupational Therapy, Elborn College Room #2539, University of Western Ontario, London, Ontario, Canada, N6G 1H1 (E-mail: jjutai@uwo.ca).

The authors gratefully acknowledge the residents and staff of Bridgepoint Health, Toronto, ON, Canada for their support of this research project.

Dr. Jutai's PIADS research program gratefully acknowledges financial support from the Ontario Ministry of Health and Long-term Care (through the Ontario Rehabilitation Technology Consortium), and the National Institute on Disability and Rehabilitation Research (through the Consortium for Assistive Technology Outcomes Research).

Copies of the PIADS questionnaire and manual may be obtained by contacting Jeffrey Jutai (*jjutai@uwo.ca*).

[Haworth co-indexing entry note]: "The Effect of Wheelchair Use on the Quality of Life of Persons with Multiple Sclerosis." Devitt, Rachel, Betty Chau, and Jeffrey W. Jutai. Co-published simultaneously in *Occupational Therapy in Health Care* (The Haworth Press, Inc.) Vol. 17, No. 3/4, 2003, pp. 63-79; and: *Occupational Therapy Practice and Research with Persons with Multiple Sclerosis* (ed: Marcia Finlayson) The Haworth Press, Inc., 2003, pp. 63-79. Single or multiple copies of this article are available for a fee from The Haworth Document Delivery Service [1-800-HAWORTH, 9:00 a.m. - 5:00 p.m. (EST). E-mail address: docdelivery@haworthpress.com].

http://www.haworthpress.com/store/product.asp?sku=J003
10.1300/J003v17n03_05

(PIADS) as an outcome measure for use by occupational therapists. Sixteen hospitalized adults with MS were interviewed using the PIADS. Descriptive comparisons of PIADS subscale scores (competence, adaptability, self-esteem) were conducted for participants using different types of wheelchairs, daily versus non-daily wheelchair users, and participants who required different levels of assistance to propel their wheelchairs. Results suggest that using a wheelchair has a positive impact on the quality of life of persons with MS. The PIADS was found to be clinically useful for exploring person-environment interactions and appears to be well suited to the goals and values of occupational therapy. Recommendations for future research and for incorporating the PIADS into occupational therapy practice are discussed. *[Article copies available for a fee from The Haworth Document Delivery Service: 1-800-HAWORTH. E-mail address: <docdelivery@haworthpress.com> Website: <http://www.HaworthPress.com> © 2003 by The Haworth Press, Inc. All rights reserved.]*

KEYWORDS. Multiple sclerosis, occupational therapy, outcome measures, Psychosocial Impact of Assistive Devices Scale (PIADS)

INTRODUCTION

Multiple sclerosis (MS) is a chronic neurological disease that can affect all aspects of a person's functioning. For example, common symptoms such as spasticity, incoordination and paralysis (Blake & Bodine, 2002) can contribute to problems with physical function, which may then lead to the use of assistive devices. In fact, mobility aids, such as wheelchairs, have been found to be the most commonly reported types of assistive devices in the possession of persons with MS (Finlayson, Guglielmello, & Liefer, 2001).

The terms assistive device and assistive technology are often used interchangeably in the literature. Adaptive or assistive technologies ". . . help an individual support their functional independence by enhancing or assisting performance in a functional activity . . ." (Smith, 1991, p. 749). For the purpose of this paper, the term assistive device will be used. Assistive devices can include low technology items such as canes and bath benches or high technology items such as power wheelchairs and electronic aids to daily living.

Research has shown that assistive devices enhance the quality of life and function of persons with disabilities (Davies, De Souza & Frank,

2003; Gryfe & Jutai, 1998; Jutai, 1999; Scherer, 1996); however, this assumption has rarely been explored in research related to persons with MS. One study by Ford, Gerry, Johnson and Tennant (2001) found that wheelchair use was a significant predictor of better quality of life in a sample of 203 persons with MS. However, the majority of research on the use and impact of assistive devices tends to focus on older adults and persons with disabilities such as spinal cord injury, stroke, brain injury, and amputations (Bender-Pape, Kim, & Weiner, 2002). Research addressing the impact of assistive devices, in particular wheelchairs, on persons with MS is important for several reasons.

First, mobility aids, such as wheelchairs, were the most frequently abandoned device category among a sample of 227 adults with chronic disabilities (Phillips & Zhao, 1993). Predictors of assistive device abandonment included lack of consideration of the device user's opinion, change in the device user's needs, and poor device performance (Phillips & Zhao). Although this study was not specific to persons with MS (i.e., 46 out of the 227 participants had MS), the findings are still valuable in that they shed some light into the reasons for device abandonment. Consequences of device abandonment may include the loss of functional abilities of the user, increases in attendant and other care costs, and ineffective use of funds from provider organizations (Day, Jutai, & Campbell, 2002; Jutai, 1999; Scherer, 1998). Further investigation of the effect of wheelchair use on persons with MS may provide additional insight into the reasons for device abandonment.

Second, additional outcomes research in the area of assistive devices, especially for costly devices such as power wheelchairs is needed (Fuhrer, 2001; Miles-Tapping & McDonald, 1994). According to Baum (1998), rehabilitation has traditionally evaluated outcomes at the level of impairment or disability. For instance, outcomes typically measured in the prescription of wheelchairs tend to address physical components such as postural control, pressure relief and sitting tolerance. However, in occupational therapy, outcomes are increasingly being measured in terms of quality of life and occupational performance (Law, Baum, & Dunn, 2001). Outcome measurement in the areas of quality of life and occupational performance can be used to document the 'real life' benefits of wheelchairs for the user. For individuals with MS, it may be particularly important to address these 'real life' quality of life outcomes because the chronic and progressive nature of the disease has been found to negatively affect quality of life (Aronson, 1997; Pfennings et al., 1999). Indeed, some authors recommend that quality of life should be used as a measure of success in assessing the impact of any assistive device intervention (Kemp, 1999).

Finally, a better understanding of the effect of wheelchair use on quality of life can support occupational therapists clinical reasoning and decision making when providing services to persons with MS. Occupational therapists play a key role in the assessment and provision of wheelchairs to persons with MS. Since wheelchairs appear to be one of the most commonly owned devices by persons with MS, therapists need to consistently measure the outcomes of their wheelchair prescriptions with this population. Measuring quality of life outcomes may provide occupational therapists with important information that helps to facilitate a better match between the needs of the client and the wheelchair.

Although there are numerous quality of life measurement scales, many are medically oriented and are designed to measure health-related quality of life, whereas most assistive devices are intended to promote function, not health per se (Jutai, 1999). In order to address this gap, Day and Jutai (1996) developed the Psychosocial Impact of Assistive Devices Scale (PIADS). The PIADS was specifically designed to measure the impact of assistive devices on the quality of life of their users and can be used to help predict the retention or abandonment of assistive devices (Jutai & Day, 2002). In a study designed to investigate the psychometric properties of a French-Canadian translation of the instrument, Demers, Monette, Descent, Jutai, and Wolfson (2002; see also Demers, Monette, Lapierrre, Arnold, & Wolfson, 2002) reported the PIADS scores from a sample of 83 persons with MS who used mobility devices such as manual and powered wheelchairs. Apart from noting that the mean scores from this sample appeared to be lower (indicating a smaller, though positive impact) than scores from a sample of clients who used vision aids, this study did not examine whether PIADS scores varied as a function of the type of wheelchair used, the frequency of device use, or the level of independence with wheelchair propulsion. Preliminary research using the PIADS suggests that device options such as tilt and power mobility may directly affect the quality of life of persons with Amyotrophic Lateral Sclerosis (ALS) (Gryfe & Jutai, 1998). However, further research is required to explore whether factors, such as the type of wheelchair used, have an effect on the quality of life of persons with MS.

The primary purpose of this pilot study was to explore the impact of wheelchair use on the quality of life of persons with MS using the PIADS. A secondary aim of the study was to examine the clinical utility of the PIADS as an assessment tool for use with clients with MS within a hospital-based seating clinic.

METHOD

Participants

A convenience sample was recruited from the neurodegenerative disorder unit of a complex continuing care hospital. Complex continuing care hospitals tend to serve a more severely functionally impaired, clinically complex population than nursing homes (Hirdes, Frijters, & Teare, 2003). The inclusion criteria consisted of a confirmed diagnosis of MS and use of a manual or power wheelchair that was either loaned or privately owned. Proxies were recruited for participants who were unable to understand and communicate responses to the study questions. Participants who did not speak English were eligible for the study if an appropriate interpreter could be arranged. Candidates were excluded from the study if they were not medically stable as determined by the unit physician. Twenty out of a potential of 22 individuals met the inclusion criteria for the study. The final sample consisted of sixteen participants (6 males and 10 females), with caregivers acting as proxies for 5 of the 16 participants. Reasons for exclusion or non-participation were owing to an inability to contact a caregiver to act as a proxy (n = 2), medical instability (n = 1), denial of the diagnosis of MS (n = 1), and not currently using a wheelchair (n = 2). The hospital ethics committee approved the study and informed consent was obtained from all participants.

Outcome Measure

The PIADS is a self-report measure that evaluates the impact of assistive devices on the quality of life of their users. According to the developers of the PIADS, "an assistive device should promote good quality of life for the user to the extent to which it makes the user feel competent, confident, and inclined (or motivated) to exploit life's possibilities" (Day et al., 2002, p. 34). These concepts of competence, confidence and inclination or motivation have been operationalized by the developers to form three subscales that are considered indices of quality of life. For a detailed discussion of how the developers conceptualized quality of life for the PIADS refer to Day et al. (2002). In brief, the first subscale, Competence, includes 12 items and measures the perceived impacts of a device on functional independence, performance and productivity. The second subscale, Self-esteem, consists of 8 items and measures the extent to which a device has affected self-confidence, self-esteem and emotional well-being. The final subscale, Adaptability, includes 6 items and measures the enabling and liberating effects of the device. Each item on all subscales is measured on a seven point scale, ranging from -3 (maximum negative impact) to $+3$ (maximum positive impact). Zero represents no change or no perceived impact because of using the device.

Past research using the PIADS has examined the impact of eyeglasses, contact lenses, hearing aids, wheelchairs, voice-output communications aids, and writing aids on the quality of life of their users (Day & Jutai, 1996; Gryfe & Jutai, 1998; Jutai, 1999; Jutai & Day, 2002). The PIADS has also been used to measure the impact of assistive device use on persons with ALS, muscular dystrophy, brain injury, spinal cord injury, and MS. It has established content validity, discriminant validity and internal reliability (Day et al., 2002). The reader is referred to Day et al. (2002) for a detailed history of the psychometric development of the PIADS.

The PIADS manual includes a Background Form for Wheelchairs that can be used to collect demographic, clinical and service-related information that might be helpful in interpreting the results from a PIADS assessment. This Form includes questions regarding the type of wheelchair, how the wheelchair is accessed or controlled, the amount of time the wheelchair is used, when the wheelchair was obtained, and satisfaction ratings. Information gathered with the Background Form can be used for both research and clinical applications. There is also a Caregiver Version of the PIADS, designed to be administered to proxies.

Procedure

The PIADS and Background Forms were administered to participants in-person by a trained interviewer. As a result of scheduling and transportation difficulties, the PIADS and Background Form were administered over the phone to 3 of the 5 proxies. One participant with expressive communication deficits communicated responses using an augmentative communication device (alphabet board). The questionnaires were also administered to one proxy in Cantonese through an interpreter. Information on the type of wheelchair and when the wheelchair was obtained was gathered from medical records, with the participant's consent, when participants were unable to provide this information.

To explore the utility and feasibility of using the PIADS with clients with MS, two occupational therapists from the hospital's seating clinic were interviewed using a set of 10 structured interview questions developed for the purpose of this study. Impressions of the interviewer were also recorded after administering the PIADS to the 16 study participants. This exploration focused on three main topics: Ease of administering, scoring and interpreting the PIADS, including its suitability for use with clients with MS; strategies for incorporating the PIADS into the seating clinic; and how findings from the PIADS may influence the wheelchair assessment and prescription process.

Analysis

Descriptive statistics, including mean, median, standard deviation, range, frequency and percentage were used to describe the participants and to perform preliminary analyses of differences in the three PIADS subscales across type of wheelchair used, frequency of wheelchair use and level of independence with wheelchair propulsion.

RESULTS

Background Form Information

The mean age of participants who completed the PIADS was 53.4 years (range 41-70). Nine participants used manual wheelchairs and seven used power wheelchairs. Participants had their current wheelchairs for a median of 42 months (range 2 weeks-10 years). Nine participants used their chair everyday for most of the day, 2 everyday for part of the day, and 5 for several days a week for part of the day.

The majority (n = 13) of participants rated the wheelchair as being extremely important to their life. Overall, participants reported a high level of satisfaction with their wheelchairs (Table 1). Participants who were independent with wheelchair propulsion gave an average satisfaction rating of 4.8 on a 5-point scale, whereas participants who required someone else to push the wheelchair for them rated their satisfaction as 2.8. (Table 2). A rating of 1 represents not satisfied and a rating of 5 represents extremely satisfied. When provided with a list of seven possible reasons for wheelchair use, 16 participants selected the main reason, as "it's the only way I can get around" and 11 of participants cited "it's the only way I can be independent." Reasons cited less frequently included increasing sitting tolerance (n = 3) and relieving pain (n = 1) (Table 3). Participants could choose all reasons that applied from the list of seven options.

PIADS Results

The mean PIADS scores were 1.54 (SD = 0.85, range 0.1 to 2.8) for the Competence subscale, 1.64 (SD = 0.82, range 0.2 to 3.0) for the Adaptability subscale, and 1.06 (SD = 0.78, range −0.4 to 2.4) for the Self-esteem subscale. Figure 1 shows subscale scores divided by different types of wheelchairs. Included in the "manual" category were participants with manual wheelchairs with no tilt. The "manual tilt" category included participants with manual wheelchairs with dynamic tilt. The "power" category included participants with power chairs with or without tilt. For participants in the "manual" category PIADS subscales were 1.1 (Competence), 1.5 (Adaptability) and 0.8 (Self-esteem). Subscale scores were 1.6 (Competence), 1.5 (Adaptability) and 1.0 (Self-esteem) for participants in the "manual tilt" category. Subscale scores for participants in the "power" category were 1.9 (Competence), 1.8 (Adaptability) and 1.3 (Self-esteem).

Figure 2 shows the mean PIADS scores between daily and non-daily users. Included in the "not everyday" category were participants who used their chairs several days a week for part of the day whereas participants who used their chairs everyday, for most or part of the day, were included in the "everyday" category. Participants in the "not everyday" category reported mean scores of below 1 on all three subscales, whereas participants in the "everyday" category reported mean scores of above 1

TABLE 1. Participant's Satisfaction with Wheelchair by Frequency of Use

Rating	Overall Satisfaction (n =15)*	Everyday (n =11)	Not Everyday (n = 4)
1	0	0	0
2	3	1	2
3	1	1	0
4	3	2	1
5	8	7	1

Note: rating of 1 represents not satisfied and rating of 5 represents extremely satisfied
*1 participant did not provide a response

TABLE 2. Wheelchair Satisfaction Ratings by Amount of Assistance Needed to Propel Chair

Amount of Assistance	Number of participants in each rating					Average rating
	1	2	3	4	5	
Someone else pushes (n = 5)	0	3	1	1	0	2.8/5
Needs some assistance (n = 3)	0	1	0	0	2	4.0/5
Independent (n = 8)	0	0	0	2	6	4.8/5

Note: rating of 1 represents not satisfied and rating of 5 represents extremely satisfied

TABLE 3. Reasons for Wheelchair Use

Reason	n
It's the only way I can get around	16
It's the only way I can be independent	11
It's the only way to approach someone	6
Because it increases my sitting tolerance	3
So that I feel less anxious	3
Because it relieves my pain	1
So that I feel less self-conscious	1
Other: because I can't tolerate being in bed	1

Note: Participants chose all reasons that applied (n =16)

FIGURE 1. Comparison of Mean PIADS Scores Among Participants Using Different Classes of Wheelchairs

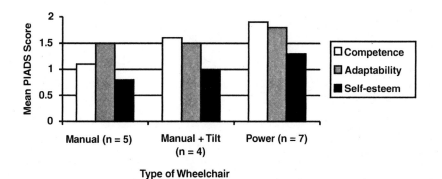

FIGURE 2. Comparison of Mean PIADS Scores Among Daily and Non-daily Users

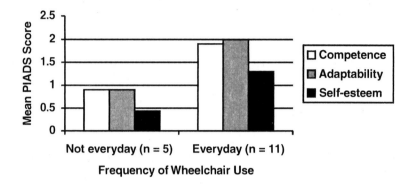

FIGURE 3. Comparison of Mean PIADS Scores Among Participants Who Need Different Levels of Assistance to Propel Chair

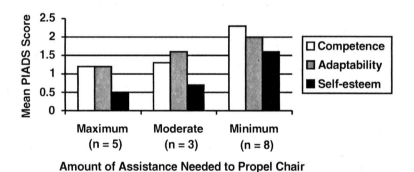

Max: participant dependent on someone else to push chair
Mod: participant occasionally needs assistance to push chair
Min: participant propels wheelchair independently

on all three subscales. PIADS subscale scores were also considered for participants who needed different levels of assistance to propel their wheelchairs (Figure 3). Included in the "maximum" category were participants who required someone to push their wheelchairs. Participants in the "moderate" category required occasional assistance to propel their wheelchairs; for example, they may have reported needing assistance when traveling longer distances. Included in the "minimum" category were participants who could independently propel their wheelchairs the majority of the time. Participants in the "maximum" and "moderate" categories had mean scores of less than 2 on the Competency and Adaptation subscales, whereas participants in the "minimum" category had mean scores of 2 or greater on the same two subscales. For the Self-esteem subscale, participants requiring moderate or maximum assistance had mean scores of below 1, whereas participants requiring minimum assistance had mean scores of above 1.

DISCUSSION

This study explored the impact of wheelchairs on the quality of life of persons with MS. A secondary aim was to evaluate the clinical utility of the PIADS as an outcome measure for use with persons with MS.

Preliminary results from the PIADS demonstrate that wheelchairs appear to have a positive impact on the perceived quality of life of persons with MS. Across the three PIADS subscales, the mean scores from the present study range from 1.06 to 1.64 and are similar to those reported by Demers, Monette, Lapierre et al. (2002) in a sample of persons with MS using mobility devices. Patterns across subscale scores are also similar to those reported in the literature involving different kinds of assistive devices across mixed diagnostic groups (Jutai, 1999). For example, preliminary results from the present study indicate that Self-esteem subscale scores are rated below Competence and Adaptability subscale scores. The Self-esteem subscale score was also the lowest score in studies on wheelchairs reported by Jutai for persons with ALS and Demers, Monette, Lapierre et al. for persons with MS. Perhaps self-esteem is affected to a large extent in degenerative diseases like MS because of the unpredictable and relapsing-remitting nature of the disease. In addition, wheelchairs may have a certain stigma attached to them (compared to assistive devices such as writing aids) which may have a subsequent negative impact on the self-esteem component of quality of life (Jutai).

There may also be an association between the length of time a device is used and the Competence subscale findings. For instance, Day and Jutai (1996) suggest that the longer an assistive device is used, the more it may contribute to feelings of competence. A similar pattern of results for the PIADS has been reported for hearing aid users (Jutai & Saunders, 2001). Participants in the present study had used their current wheelchairs on average for a median of 42 months, which may have contributed to their positive perceptions of competence. However, because of an insufficient sample size, correlations between subscale scores and variables such as length of time using a wheelchair were not examined in this study.

The Adaptability subscale score was rated the highest of all subscale scores and this is similar to results found by Demers, Monette, Lapierre et al. (2002) in a sample of persons with MS using mobility aids and by Gryfe and Jutai (1998) in a sample of persons with ALS using wheelchairs. This finding highlights the importance of focusing on domains of adaptation, such as how using a wheelchair affects a person's ability to participate and to adapt to new things, in addition to the physical aspects of functioning in the assessment and provision of wheelchairs

Preliminary findings also suggest that wheelchair options such as the addition of tilt and power mobility may impact positively on quality of life. This finding is similar to results obtained by Gryfe and Jutai (1998) in a sample of persons with ALS. The impact on quality of life for persons with ALS increased significantly with the devices' capabilities for powered mobility and postural adjustment. Perhaps these options allow participants to stay longer in their chairs, conserve energy, access a variety of environments (Miles-Tapping & MacDonald, 1994) and participate in more occupations throughout the day.

It appears that being able to move about in a wheelchair more independently also has a positive impact on quality of life. Average satisfaction ratings in the present study (from the PIADS Background Form) appeared to decrease as the assistance that participants required from others to propel their chairs increased. Perhaps being able to control where and when you move around allows you to have greater control over your environment, which leads to a greater perceived impact on quality of life. Future research is needed to examine variables such as the type of wheelchair, frequency of wheelchair use and independence with wheelchair mobility and their association with PIADS scores in persons with MS.

Clinical Utility of the PIADS

Findings from the structured interview with the two occupational therapists in the seating clinic and the impressions of the interviewer after administering the PIADS to the study participants appear to confirm the clinical utility of the PIADS. Several interesting issues were explored that lend themselves to further discussion. First, with respect to ease of administration, the PIADS and Background Form for each participant in this study required approximately 25 minutes to complete.

The PIADS questionnaire itself took no more·than 5 minutes to score. The checklist format of the PIADS and Background Form allowed information to be recorded easily and the final scores to be presented graphically, which made the results easier to understand and explain to others. These factors contributed positively to the feasibility of incorporating the PIADS into practice.

Second, the suitability of administering the PIADS with persons with MS was explored. Although the manual states that the PIADS can be used with varied diagnostic groups, observations from this study revealed that good cognitive abilities are needed to comprehend the meanings of the items in the scale, to reflect on the meanings, and to assign a rating. For instance, terms such as 'skillfulness' and 'adequacy' were difficult for some participants to comprehend, even when provided with an explanation from the glossary in the PIADS manual. If cognitive impairment is significant enough to limit administration of the PIADS, the Caregiver (proxy) Version of the PIADS is a good alternative and may allow a more diverse population to be included in research studies and clinical applications. Although research has shown that a proxy completing the PIADS is a valid measure of the impact of assistive devices on the user's quality of life (Jutai, Woolrich, Campbell, Gryfe, & Day, 2000), this appears to be an area of some debate in the literature. For example, research has found that participant-proxy agreement is greater on objective rather than subjective measures and that proxies tend to underestimate quality of life (Andresen, Vahle, & Lollar, 2001). However, the use of proxy report may be unavoidable in some situations in order that client-centered measures can be obtained.

Recommendations for Incorporating the PIADS into OT Practice

The two occupational therapists interviewed felt that the PIADS could be included during the initial seating clinic assessment and at subsequent follow-up periods to provide information on the impact of the wheelchair over time. However, several factors play a key role in the successful incorporation of outcome measures such as the PIADS into occupational therapy practice. Ideally, there needs to be the support and shared commitment of an organization or hospital to examining the outcomes of occupational therapy service efforts (Jutai, Ladak, Schuller, Naumann, & Wright, 1996). Occupational therapists also need to have the skills and time to investigate, select and introduce new outcome measures into their services. This can be accomplished through carrying out collaborative research such as in this study, which allowed practicing occupational therapists to become actively involved in the process of evaluating and exploring the PIADS.

The process of deciding how to implement the PIADS into practice needs to be linked to clients' goals and to the values of the profession of occupational therapy. For clients with degenerative illnesses such as MS, goals are often related to maintaining or enhancing occupational performance and quality of life. This linking can be achieved through employing occupation-based models such as the Person-Environment-Occupation Model (PEO) (Law et al., 1996) and additional assessments such as The Canadian Occupational Performance Measure (COPM) (Law et al., 1998) in the process of assessing and prescribing wheelchairs. For example, using the PEO Model, the wheelchair can be viewed as an extension of the external physical environment in interaction with the person and his or her occupations. The outcome of this interaction can have an enabling or constraining influence on both occupational performance and quality of life. The PIADS allows for the exploration of person-environment interactions and appears to be well suited to the underlying concepts of the PEO Model. Linking the PIADS with occupational therapy practice models such as the PEO would ensure that the individual's occupations are also considered in the design or selection of wheelchairs.

Findings from the PIADS can influence the wheelchair assessment and prescription process in several ways. Incorporating the PIADS into the assessment process would enhance client-centered practice by increasing the focus on important quality of life outcomes in addition to traditional performance component outcomes such as pressure mapping and postural alignment. The PIADS would also stimulate discussion of psychosocial issues and highlight problematic areas. For instance, if a particular type of wheelchair had a negative impact on domains of quality of life, an alternative wheelchair could be explored and potential device abandonment may be avoided. The PIADS could also help validate that wheelchairs help people with MS function and ". . . allow them to adapt or cope better with their disease" (Gryfe & Jutai, 1998, p. 30). Furthermore, the PIADS could be used to facilitate collaborative goal setting and discussion on the quality of life impact of the assistive device in relation to the importance and functional significance of the areas identified in the subscales (Day, Jutai, Woolrich, & Strong, 2001).

Several limitations must be considered when interpreting the findings from this study. Generalization of the results is limited by the use of a small convenience sample and the lack of more detailed demographic data. As such, the findings should only be considered as exploratory and preliminary. The variable length of time of wheelchair use (2 weeks to 10 years) in this study could have influenced the results. It is also important to keep in mind that factors such as depression or cognitive deficits, which were not measured as part of this study, could have influenced study results. Specifically, Fruehwald, Loeffler-Stastka, Eher, Saletu, and Baumhackl (2001) recommend using a screening instrument in studies to help detect depressive disorders in MS and their influence on self-assessed quality. Future research using the PIADS with persons with MS could include screening instruments as recommended by Fruehwald et al.

It is also important to understand that the concept of quality of life is multidimensional and that the PIADS is not claiming to be a comprehensive measure of quality of life outcomes related to assistive devices. Instead, it should be kept in mind that the PIADS captures information on important domains of quality of life that matter to the users of these devices. Nonetheless, it is very encouraging that the findings from the small sample in this study appear to be quite consistent with results from other independent investigations using the PIADS with clients who have MS (Demers, Monette, Lapierre et al., 2002). This suggests that the patterns of PIADS scores might be predictably associated with specific clinical populations of assistive device users (Jutai, 1999).

CONCLUSION

In conclusion, preliminary findings reveal that wheelchair use appears to have a positive impact on the quality of life of persons with MS. The process of selecting a wheelchair is complex for persons with MS and their health care providers and it is made even more complex by the huge selection of wheelchair models, backs, seat cushions, and accessories available on the market. The PIADS can assist with this complex process particularly when used in combination with relevant models of practice, occupation-based assessments, and with assessments that are focused on matching the person's physical abilities to the wheelchair. A structured approach to determining the impact of wheelchairs on the quality of life of persons with MS, combined with a consideration of the person's occupational performance, will result in an approach that best meets the needs of clients with MS and the values and goals of the profession of occupational therapy.

REFERENCES

Andresen, E., Vahle, V.J., & Lollar, D. (2001). Proxy reliability: Health-related quality of life (HRQoL) measures for people with disability. *Quality of Life Research, 10*(7), 609-619.

Aronson, K. J. (1997). Quality of life among persons with multiple sclerosis and their caregivers. *Neurology, 48*(1), 74-80.

Baum, C. (1998). Achieving effectiveness with a client-centered approach: A person-environment interaction. In D.B. Gray, L.A. Quatrano, & L. Lieberman (Eds.), *Designing and Using Assistive Technology: The Human Perspective* (pp. 137-147). Baltimore, MD: Paul H. Brooks Publishing Company

Bender-Pape, T.L., Kim, J., & Weiner, B. (2002). The shaping of individual meanings assigned to assistive technology: A review of personal factors. *Disability and Rehabilitation, 24*(1-3), 5-20.

Blake, D.J. & Bodine, C. (2002). An overview of assistive technology for persons with multiple sclerosis. *Journal of Rehabilitation Research and Development, 39*(2), 299-312.

Day, H., & Jutai, J. (1996). Measuring the Psychosocial Impact of Assistive Devices: The PIADS. *Canadian Journal of Rehabilitation, 9*(3), 159-168.

Day, H. Jutai, J., & Campbell, K.A. (2002). Development of a scale to measure the psychosocial impact of assistive devices: Lessons learned and the road ahead. *Disability and Rehabilitation, 24*(1-3), 31-37.

Day, H., Jutai, J., Woolrich, W., & Strong, G. (2001). The stability of impact of assistive devices. *Disability and Rehabilitation, 23*(9), 400-404.

Davies, A., De Souza, L.H., & Frank, A.O. (2003). Changes in the quality of life of severely disabled people following provision of powered indoor/outdoor chairs. *Disability and Rehabilitation, 25*, 286-290.

Demers, L., Monette, M., Descent, M., Jutai, J., & Wolfson, C. (2002). The Psychosocial Impact of Assistive Devices Scale (PIADS): Translation and preliminary psychometric evaluation of a Canadian-French version. *Quality of Life Research, 11*(6), 583-592.

Demers, L., Monette, M., Lapierre, Y., Arnold, D.L., & Wolfson, C. (2002). Reliability, validity, and applicability of the Quebec User Evaluation of Satisfaction with Assistive Technology (QUEST 2.0) for adults with multiple sclerosis. *Disability and Rehabilitation, 24*(1-3), 21-30.

Finlayson, M., Guglielmello, L., & Liefer, K. (2001). Describing and predicting the possession of assistive devices among persons with multiple sclerosis. *The American Journal of Occupational Therapy, 55*(5), 545-551.

Ford, H.L., Gerry, E., Johnson, M.H., & Tennant, A. (2001). Health status and quality of life of people with multiple sclerosis. *Disability and Rehabilitation, 23*(12), 516-521.

Fruehwald, S., Loeffler-Stastka, H., Eher, H.,Saletu, B., & Baumhackl, U. (2001). Depression and quality of life in multiple sclerosis. *Acta Neurologica Scandinavica, 104*(5), 257-261.

Fuhrer, M.J. (2001). Assistive technology outcomes research: Challenges met and yet unmet. *American Journal of Physical Medicine and Rehabilitation, 80*(7), 528-535.

Gryfe, P. & Jutai, J. (1998). Assistive technologies: Clients' perceptions of impact on quality of life. *Rehab and Community Care Management, 7,* 26-30.

Hirdes, J.P., Frijters, D.H., & Teare, G.F. (2003). The MDS-CHESS Scale: A new measure to predict mortality in institutionalized older people. *Journal of the American Geriatrics Society, 51,* 96-100.

Jutai, J. (1999). Quality of life impact of assistive technology. *Rehabilitation Engineering, 14,* 2-7.

Jutai, J. & Day, H. (2002). Psychosocial Impact of Assistive Devices Scale (PIADS). *Technology and Disability, 14,* 107-111.

Jutai, J., Ladak, N., Schuller, R., Naumann, S., & Wright, V. (1996). Outcomes measurement of assistive technologies: An institutional case study. *Assistive Technology, 8*(2), 110-120.

Jutai, J. & Saunders, G. (2001). Psychosocial impact of hearing aids with a generic scale. American Academy of Audiology, San Diego, California, April 19-22.

Jutai, J., Woolrich, W., Campbell, K., Gryfe, P., & Day, H. (2000). User-caregiver agreement on perceived psychosocial impact of assistive devices. Proceedings of RESNA 2000, Orlando, Florida, 328-330.

Kemp, B. J. (1999). Quality of life while aging with a disability. *Assistive Technology, 11*(2), 158-163.

Law, M., Baptiste, S., Carswell, A., McColl, M.A., Polatajko, H., & Pollock, N. (1998). *Canadian Occupational Performance Measure* (3rd ed.). Ottawa, ON: Canadian Association of Occupational Therapists.

Law, M., Baum, C., & Dunn, W. (2001). Measuring occupational performance: Supporting best practice in occupational therapy. Thorofare, NJ: SLACK Incorporated.

Law, M., Cooper, B.A., Strong, S., Stewart, D., Rigby, P., & Letts, L. (1996). The Person-Environment-Occupation Model: A transactive approach to occupational performance. *Canadian Journal of Occupational Therapy, 63*(1), 9-23.

Miles-Tapping, C. & MacDonald, L.J. (1994). Lifestyle implications of power mobility . . . electric wheelchair and scooter users. *Physical & Occupational Therapy in Geriatrics, 12*(4), 31-49.

Pfennings, L., Cohen, L., Ader, H., Polman, C., Lankhurst, G., Smits, R., & van der Ploeg, H. (1999). Exploring differences between subgroups of multiple sclerosis patients in health-related quality of life. *Journal of Neurology, 246*(7), 587-591.

Phillips, B., & Zhao, H. (1993). Predictors of assistive technology abandonment. *Assistive Technology, 5*(1), 36-45.

Scherer, M.J. (1996). Outcomes of assistive technology use on quality of life. *Disability and Rehabilitation, 18*(9), 439-448.

Scherer, M.J. (1998). The impact of assistive technology on the lives of people with disabilities. In D.B. Gray, L.A. Quatrano, & L. Lieberman (Eds.), *Designing and Using Assistive Technology: The Human Perspective* (pp. 99-115). Baltimore, MD: Paul H. Brooks Publishing Company.

Scherer, M. & Galvin, J.C. (1994). Matching people with technology. *Rehab Management: The Interdisciplinary Journal of Rehabilitation, 7*(2), 128-130.

Smith, R.O. (1991). Technological approaches to performance enhancement. In. C. Christiansen & C. Baum (Eds.), *Occupational Therapy: Overcoming Human Performance Deficits* (pp. 748-786). Thorofare, NJ: SLACK Incorporated.

Interference of Upper Limb Tremor on Daily Life Activities in People with Multiple Sclerosis

Peter Feys, PT, PhD student
Anders Romberg, PT
Juhnai Ruutiainen, MD
Pierre Ketelaer, MD

SUMMARY. The interference of upper limb intention tremor on activities of daily living was described in 32 persons with multiple sclerosis. Ratings about their degree of impairment and disability (Functional Systems, Expanded Disability Status Scale, Functional Independence Measure) was obtained from the multidisciplinary rehabilitation team. The individuals were interviewed using a questionnaire, mainly based on the

---

Peter Feys is a PhD student, Faculty of Physical Education and Physiotherapy, Department of Kinesiology, Tervuursevest 101, 3001 Leuven, Belgium (E-mail: Peter.Feys@flok.kuleuven.ac.be).

Anders Romberg is affiliated with the Masku Neurological Rehabilitation Centre, P.O. Box 15, 21251 Masku, Finland (E-mail: anders.romberg@ms-liitto.fi).

Juhnai Ruutiainen is MS Neurologist, Masku Neurological Rehabilitation Centre, P.O. Box 15, 21251 Masku, Finland (E-mail: juhani.ruutiainen@masku.pp.fi).

Pierre Ketelaer is MS Neurologist, National Multiple Sclerosis Centre, Vanheylenstraat 16, 1820 Melsbroek, Belgium (E-mail: ms-mels@rims.be).

This study was financially supported by the TREMOR Tide Project DE3216, funded by the European Commission (DG XIII).

[Haworth co-indexing entry note]: "Interference of Upper Limb Tremor on Daily Life Activities in People with Multiple Sclerosis." Feys, Peter et al. Co-published simultaneously in *Occupational Therapy in Health Care* (The Haworth Press, Inc.) Vol. 17, No. 3/4, 2003, pp. 81-95; and: *Occupational Therapy Practice and Research with Persons with Multiple Sclerosis* (ed: Marcia Finlayson) The Haworth Press, Inc., 2003, pp. 81-95. Single or multiple copies of this article are available for a fee from The Haworth Document Delivery Service [1-800-HAWORTH, 9:00 a.m. - 5:00 p.m. (EST). E-mail address: docdelivery@haworthpress.com].

items of the FIM scale, about the interference of tremor during activities of daily life. Intention tremor is rarely an isolated symptom. It is extremely disabling and was reported to interfere the most with activities of daily life such as eating, drinking, grooming and dressing. A variety of aids and strategies to compensate for specific disabilities were reported reflecting the important counseling role of the occupational therapist in assisting persons to cope more effectively with tremor. *[Article copies available for a fee from The Haworth Document Delivery Service: 1-800-HAWORTH. E-mail address: <docdelivery@haworthpress.com> Website: <http://www.HaworthPress.com> © 2003 by The Haworth Press, Inc. All rights reserved.]*

KEYWORDS. Intention tremor, multiple sclerosis, disability, Functional Independence Measure, self-care aids

Multiple sclerosis (MS) is a disabling neurological disease affecting young adults in the United States and Northern and Central Europe. The prevalence of multiple sclerosis in such areas is estimated between 50 and 120 per 100,000 inhabitants (Ebers, 1998). Upper limb tremor is reported to occur in about one third of people with multiple sclerosis (Alusi, Glickman, Aziz, & Bain, 1999; Alusi, Worthington, Glickman, & Bain, 2001; Ruutiainen, 1997; Weinshenker, Issa, & Baskerville, 1996).

Intention tremor, as defined by the Movement Disorders Society on Tremor, is present if the amplitude of tremor increases towards the end of goal-directed movements (Deuschl, Bain, & Brin, 1998). It is commonly associated with dysfunction of the cerebellum or its connections (Alusi et al., 2001; Nakamura et al., 1993). Intention tremor is greater during visually-guided movements compared to during movement execution with the eyes closed (Liu et al., 1997). In line with its definition, intention tremor is very likely to interfere with activities of daily living such as picking up the receiver of the telephone or drinking a glass of wine. Intention tremor is still an underestimated cause of disability, perhaps because it is often part of a wider clinical picture in MS. The functional impact of tremor may be easily overlooked in conventional bedside neurological examination. However, even the mildest degree of intention tremor of the hand can disturb a person's handwriting and personal computer interaction or his abilities in drinking (Feys et al., 2001; Schenk, Walther & Mai, 2000).

Intention tremor in multiple sclerosis is rarely an isolated symptom (Alusi et al., 2001). It is frequently embedded in a complex movement disorder, which often includes dysmetria and other ataxic features (Alusi et al., 1999). In these persons with multiple sclerosis, ataxia refers to an incoordination of the movement following damage of the cerebellar system (Bastian, 1997). Cerebellar dysfunction in MS has been identified as an important factor determining rehabilitation outcome (Langdon & Thompson, 1999). The severity of ataxia (Langdon & Thompson, 1999; Weinshenker et al., 1996) and more specific tremor (Alusi et al., 1999; Matsumoto et al., 2001) correlates highly with the level of disability and dependence of the person. However, only a few quantitative studies have provided some information about the possible contribution of tremor to disabilities caused by multiple sclerosis. Alusi et al. and Matsumoto et al. used a tremor-related disability questionnaire (25 items about activities of daily life), which was originally developed and validated for the study of essential tremor (Bain et al., 1993). The participant had to rate how difficult it was to perform the activity (no, little, a lot of effort or not possible) because of the tremor. As such, however, other symptoms such as muscle weakness may interfere with the outcome scores. The same comment is applicable to the study of Jones, Lewis, Harrisson, and Wiles (1996), where subjects had to rate their performance, taking into account their tremor on the items of the Northwick Park ADL Index (Sheikh et al., 1979) using the visual analogue scales (0-100 mm, 0 = worst).

This study was part of the European TREMOR Project DE3216 (1996-1999) that focused on disability caused by upper limb intention tremor due to multiple sclerosis. The purpose of this descriptive study was to identify the needs of this group of people in more detail for reasons of specific goal setting in the development of new assistive devices for the treatment of disabilities caused by tremor. Basically, to establish the degree of (in)dependence, people with intention tremor due to MS were rated on the items of the Functional Independence Measure (FIM), which provides a comprehensive disability assessment. To establish the perceived influence of tremor during activities of daily life, these people with MS were asked to rate the interference of intention tremor during the same items of the FIM. In addition, an inventory was made of the person's aids and strategies to cope with their specific disabilities.

METHODS

Participants

Persons with upper limb intention tremor due to multiple sclerosis were selected by referral from the physician of the National Centre for

Multiple Sclerosis, Melsbroek (Belgium) or the Masku Neurological Rehabilitation Centre (Finland). The degree of intention tremor was rated with Fahn's tremor rating scale (0-4). Fahn's tremor rating scale was found to be highly reliable for rating MS tremor during the finger-to-nose test (Hooper, Taylor, Pentland, & Whittle, 1998) and is commonly used in studies dealing with intention tremor (Deuschl, Wenzelburger, Loffler, Raethjen, & Stolze, 2000; Feys, Duportail, Kos, Van Asch, & Ketelaer, 2002; Feys et al., 2003b; Niranjan, Kondziolka, Baser, Heyman, & Lunsford, 2000).

Exclusion criteria were an Expanded Disability Status Scale (EDSS) score (Kurtzke, 1983) more than 8.5 (i.e., restricted to the bed most of the day without effective use of the arms) and a score lower than 24 on the Mini Mental State Examination (MMSE) (0-30) (Beatty & Goodkin, 1990; Folstein et al., 1975). The former criterion was added to select only persons with some effective use of their arms that was not influenced by bed positioning. The latter criterion was used to interview only persons with relatively preserved cognitive function for reasonably answering of questions. The EDSS and MMSE were administered by the physician.

Data Collection and Procedures

Standard Scales. The degree of impairment and disability was obtained from the medical notes of each person. The Functional Systems (FS) (Kurtzke, 1983), rated by the physician, provides information on impairment of the pyramidal, cerebellar, sensory, bowel and bladder, brain stem, visual and mental system of the person (0-5 rating scale for each item, except of pyramidal system: 0-6).

The Functional Independence Measure (FIM) (Linacre, Heinemann, Wright, Granger, & Hamilton, 1994), rated by the different members of the rehabilitation team, is an 18-item scale which rates the level of assistance required to perform various activities of daily living using a seven-level scoring system. The FIM provides information about activities such as mobility, self-care, communication, etc. The FIM is commonly used in MS rehabilitation settings and has been shown to be reliable and sensitive to change (Granger, Cotter, Hamilton, Fiedler, & Hens, 1990; Jones et al., 1996; Sharrack, Hughes, Soudain, & Dunn, 1999). Two items of the FIM (comprehension and memory) were not included in this study as the interference of tremor is difficult to estimate for these items.

Survey. All participants were interviewed by a researcher (one in each center), who was familiar with persons with MS who have tremor.

The interview guide was a structured instrument developed by the researchers of the TREMOR project and was always completed within one hour. The participants were asked to appraise the perceived degree of interference of tremor (none, mild, marked or severe) for the above-mentioned items of the FIM and to report any possible aid or strategy to compensate for the specific disability. In addition, the researcher asked during the structured interview if tremor interfered during four specific functional activities (shaving or applying make-up, picking up a pen, handwriting, operating a remote control) and during household and recreational activities.

Informed consent was obtained from all participants. The study was conducted in agreement with the 1964 Declaration of Helsinki and approved by the local ethics committee.

Data Analysis

Descriptive statistics were used throughout. Mean and standard deviation or median and range were calculated to describe the characteristics and ratings of the participants. Furthermore, the number and percentage of persons in a specific category (FS) or reporting a specific interference of tremor was determined.

RESULTS

Participants

Thirty-two persons with upper limb intention tremor due to multiple sclerosis were included in this pilot study. Eighteen and 14 persons respectively were selected from the National Centre for Multiple Sclerosis, Melsbroek (Belgium) and the Masku Neurological Rehabilitation Centre (Finland). All participants showed mild to marked intention tremor during the finger-to-nose test (Feys et al., 2003b) as rated with Fahn's tremor rating scale (0-4). One quarter of the group had unilateral intention tremor whereas all the other showed bilateral intention tremor. Thirteen participants were male and nineteen were female. Average age was 44.3 years (SD 10.1) ranging from 30 to 65. The mean duration of the disease was 13.9 years (SD 6.9). The median EDSS score was 7.25 with range 6.0-8.5, which indicated that all participants needed constant unilateral or bilateral assistance to walk or were restricted to the wheelchair most of the time. The median score on the Mini Mental Scale was

27 (range 24-30), indicating that the persons were cognitively able to reasonably answer the questions.

Findings from Standard Scales

The data of the Functional Systems are shown in Table 1. Most of the 32 people who were interviewed (84 %) had a mild paraparesis, hemiparesis or severe monoparesis. Three quarters of the sample used a wheelchair exclusively with the majority using a manual wheelchair. Two thirds of the persons showed some impairment of the eye motor control system, for example, nystagmus. Nearly one third of the persons interviewed had a normal sensory function while the other showed a mild decrease. The majority of the participants were frequently incontinent. Fifty-nine percent of the group had a normal visual acuity. Most of the participants had a normal mental function or some mood alteration only.

The median FIM score for each item and the number of participants who mentioned a moderate to severe interference of tremor during the execution of that specific activity are presented in Table 2.

The median FIM score was 6.0 for most ADL functions, which indicates that half of the group was completely independent for these activities of daily life. Exceptions were bathing, dressing upper and lower body and bladder control that showed a median FIM score of 4.0 and 4.5 respectively. This indicates that the majority of participants needed assistance for these activities.

Participant Survey Findings

The vast majority of the participants reported moderate to severe hindrance of the upper limb tremor during eating and drinking. Half of all persons experienced moderate to severe interference of tremor during grooming and dressing the upper body. The median FIM score was 1.0 for walking and stairs that implies that half the group needed full assistance. Two persons mentioned trunk ataxia while walking. Nobody was totally dependent for driving a wheelchair. Three quarters of the group experienced minimal or no interference of the tremor while driving the wheelchair. The specific aids and strategies reported by the subjects for daily life activities are shown in Table 3.

Half of the group was still capable of shaving (male) or using make-up (female). However, 69% experienced interference of tremor with the activity. A similar number of subjects felt interference of tremor while picking up a ballpoint from the table, but were still able to perform this.

TABLE 1. Median Score for the Functional Systems and Categorization of Patients

FUNCTIONAL SYSTEMS	Median	No impairment (score 0)	Mild impairment (score 1-2)	Moderate to Severe impairment (score > 3)
Pyramidal (0-6)	3	1 (3%)	4 (13%)	27 (84%)
Cerebellar (0-5)	3	0 (0%)	2 (06%)	30 (94%)
Brain Stem (0-5)	3	2 (6%)	10 (31%)	20 (63%)
Sensory (0-5)	2	10 (31%)	8 (25%)	14 (44%)
Bowel, Bladder (0-5)	2	2 (6%)	15 (47%)	15 (47%)
Visual (0-5)	0	19 (59%)	6 (19%)	7 (22%)
Mental (0-5)	1	13 (41%)	18 (56%)	1 (03%)

All systems consist of a 6 point grading scale (0-5) except for the pyramidal system (0-6).

TABLE 2. Median of FIM Scores and Number of Patients (Percentages) Reporting Moderate or Severe Interference of Tremor

FIM ITEMS	MEDIAN	MODERATE OR SEVERE INTERFERENCE OF TREMOR N = 32
EATING	6	26 (81%)
GROOMING	6	17 (53%)
DRESSING UPPER BODY	4	16 (50%)
DRESSING LOWER BODY	4.5	12 (37%)
BATHING	4	11 (34%)
TOILETING	6	11 (34%)
TRANSFER BED/CHAIR	6	10 (31%)
TRANSFER TOILET	6	10 (31%)
TRANSFER TUB/SHOWER	5	9 (28%)
WALK	1	10 (31%)
WHEELCHAIR	6	8 (25%)
STAIRS	1	8 (25%)
BOWEL	6	7 (23%)
BLADDER	4	8 (25%)
SOCIAL INTERACTION	6	5 (16%)
EXPRESSION	6	1 (03%)

FIM Levels: (Modified) Independence: 6-7 (no helper)
        Modified Dependence: 3-4-5 (helper)
        Complete Dependence: 1-2 (helper)
The degree of interference: none, mild, moderate, severe

Eighty-one percent of the subjects experienced tremor while writing, 69% were capable of writing a word although it was rather difficult for more than one quarter of the group. Most participants reported that their handwriting had deteriorated compared to the past. Some of them wrote in capital letters. Most of the subjects mentioned spontaneously that they were unable to write many sentences in succession without rest.

Ninety percent of the group was capable of operating the remote control of the television. However, the majority of them experienced interference of upper limb tremor with this activity. Some compensated for this by fixing the remote control against the trunk or by stabilizing the active hand with the other. One person remarked that the buttons of the remote control are too close to each other. Half of the group had given up hobbies or recreational activities because of intention tremor. Thirty

TABLE 3. Compensatory Aids and Strategies for Activities of Daily Life (FIM Items)

FIM ITEMS	AIDS	STRATEGIES
EATING, DRINKING	thickened and weighted cutlery and cup, plates, plastic plates, raised edge, non-skid material, weighted cuffs on wrist	drink with a straw, use of both hands, fixating elbow against trunk or table, half-filled glass, cook with microwave
GROOMING, BATHING	soap-on-a-rope, mirror for visual cueing, non-skid material, electric toothbrush	stabilize one hand with the other
DRESSING UPPER/LOWER BODY	big buttons, velcro fastenings instead of buttons or laces, a metal ring attached at the zipper, socksurrounder, a long shoelifter	loose clothing, lower buttons already closed in advance
TRANSFER BED, (WHEEL)CHAIR, TUB, SHOWER	ramps, handrails, grabbars sliding board, electric bed, raised toilet	anticipate positioning of the wheelchair, look for supplementary support, speed control
WALKING	sticks, weighted rollator, pulpit walker	fixation of hand on back, speed control, widened base of feet
WHEELCHAIR	electric wheelchair, head-rest , lateral support, safety belt, long handled brakes, weighted cuffs on wrists, non-skid material on hoopers/the wheels, spoke protectors	
STAIRS	ramps on both sides, non-skid material on steps	
EXPRESSION, COMMUNICATION	weighted cuff on wrist for writing, penholder, hand free phone, Personal Computer: slower mouse, larger screen, keyboard covered with keyguard, voice activated computers	be patient use of ice prior to conversation

percent of the subjects had adapted or changed their recreational activities. Examples of activities that were abandoned are collecting stamps, knitting, cycling, playing the guitar, drawing and writing. More than half of the persons had given up participating in household activities; one third of the subjects could adapt some activities (for example, cooking with microwave).

DISCUSSION

This study described the perceived interference of intention tremor on activities of daily life by interviewing participants having tremor due to multiple sclerosis. A clinical picture of the sample at the level of impairment and disability was provided by therapists' ratings of the Functional Systems and Functional Independence Measure.

The results on the Functional Systems, providing the picture at the level of impairment, support previous findings (Alusi et al., 2001) that upper limb tremor is rarely an isolated symptom in persons with multiple sclerosis. The presence of multiple symptoms in these persons with multiple sclerosis means that the median FIM scores must be interpreted with caution. The degree of dependence in the execution of activities of daily life can be the consequence of different symptoms. In addition, these activities do not always involve both arms to the same extent and thus, the person may compensate for specific activities with the less affected arm. Studies with larger samples that can examine the relationships between intention tremor and FIM scores using multivariate analysis would be useful in the future.

The same precautions must be kept in mind when interpreting the person's reports about interference of tremor during activities of daily life. The interference of unilateral tremor may not (or to a lesser extent) be reported if the other arm can take over. This can explain why a moderate to severe interference of tremor was mentioned only for three items of the FIM by at least the majority of participants. Another influencing factor is the inventiveness of some persons to cope with difficulties caused by tremor. It could be that those persons who made use of specific aids or strategies reported less interference of tremor than other persons did. As a consequence, the contribution of tremor with some activities is difficult to estimate precisely.

Still, the percentage of persons who indicated a moderate to severe interference of tremor while eating and drinking is high. Eating and drinking require high levels of fine motor control. Even when only one arm is impaired, cutting meat is difficult. Moreover, the threat of spilling creates a stressful situation, possibly aggravating the intention tremor (Ketola, 1995). The same is true for activities such as putting on make-up. The interference of tremor during these activities may result in making a mess and becoming soiled, which can lead to restrictions in social participation, for example, choosing to not take meals in restaurants. In the study of Alusi et al. (2001), persons with tremor reported that they felt handicapped either because of the physical effects of tremor or because they were embarrassed by the tremor, or both. The number of participants that reported giving up their household and recreational activities because of intention tremor emphasizes the effect of tremor on activity and participation.

Tremor obviously restricts the written communication of many individuals as they experience more difficulties in handwriting due to tremor. One out of three subjects was not capable of writing one readable word. Handwriting deficits are frequently encountered in MS (Wellingham-Jones, 1991) and were recently quantitatively analyzed in people with MS with cerebellar signs by means of a digitizing tablet (Schenk et al., 2000). The study concluded persons with tremor due to multiple sclerosis were capable of performing stroke movements required in handwriting. However, vision is needed to prevent letter distortions in size or form. Intention tremor is known to be enhanced when visual feedback (of movement errors) is being used (Feys et al., in press; Liu et al., 1997), explaining the reported interference of tremor during handwriting. The use of a personal computer (PC), as mentioned by some individuals as compensatory aid, may provide a solution. However, interacting with the PC by means of graphic user interfaces was also found to be difficult for many people (Feys et al., 2001). One of the achievements of the European TREMOR project was the facilitation of PC interaction by using compensatory hardware interfaces such as a trackball and/or an assistive software program that filters tremor components of the hand/interface movement (so-called tremor control system) (Feys et al., 2001).

The participants reported variable compensatory aids and strategies for the different items of the FIM. Weighted cuffs have been advocated for reduction of the amplitude of tremor (Dahlin-Webb, 1986), however, the beneficial effect seems minimal (Kraft, 1998) or even not present (Feys et al., 2003a; Morrice, Becker, Hoffer, & Lee, 1990). Because literature about compensatory aids and strategies for coping with tremor is very limited and as tremor is difficult to distinguish from ataxic features such as dysmetria, we refer to studies on ataxia as well. Adapted and weighted equipment such as cutlery are commonly recommended aids included in rehabilitation programs for ataxic persons (Gillen, 2000; Jones et al., 1996; Kraft, 1998; Yuen, 1993). Some of the compensatory aids and strategies, reported by the participants, were also discussed in studies concerning the effect of occupational therapy on activities of daily life performance in persons with ataxia (Gillen, 2000; Jones et al., 1996). For example, using weighted items (such as cutlery and walking frames), an electric toothbrush (minimization of the need to perform rapid alternating movements) or a soap-on-a-rope (decrease of manipulation demands) were presented as appropriate solutions. In the same way, the strategy to decrease the degree of freedom (number of joints) during functional activities requiring distal function, by stabilizing the upper extremities against the trunk or environment (e.g., table), was reported by both the participants and researchers (Bastian, 1997; Gillen, 2000; Jones et al., 1996). Thus, the role of the occupational therapist as counselor on compensatory aids and strategies in daily life activities is highly acknowledged, as reflected by participants' comments.

The studies by Gillen (2000) and Jones et al. (1996) demonstrated that occupational therapy programs can be effective for functionally coping with upper limb ataxia, if an individualized program of interventions, designed to meet the individual's priorities and potential, is developed. Both counseling and provision of adaptive equipment and training of adapted movement patterns (with incorporation of environment) are important (Kesselring & Thompson, 1997). Interestingly, Gillen (2000) made use of the FIM-items to evaluate performance component dysfunction and to discuss the therapy goals with the person himself. As such, the person expressed in which activities he was satisfied with his performance and in which activities interventions were desired. As the degree of tremor has been shown to be highly related to disability (Alusi et al., 2001; Langdon & Thompson, 1999; Matsumoto et al., 2001) and as adapted therapy programs have been shown to be effective in improving functional performance (Gillen, 2000; Jones et al., 1996), analysis of the interference of tremor during daily life is appropriate. For this purpose, the FIM is a good instrument, as the ratings and observations of therapists during specific daily life activities can be easily integrated with the person's rating of tremor interference. In further support of the potential effect of therapy on function in persons with ataxia, Armutlu et al. (2001) showed in their pilot study that an intensive physiotherapeutic treatment program (including weight transfer, Frenkel coordination exercises, stabilization techniques involving positioning and proprioceptive neuromuscular facilitation) improved balance and walking.

CONCLUSION

Intention tremor is rarely an isolated symptom in multiple sclerosis, but is a very important cause of disability. Tremor is perceived to interfere the most with activities of daily life such as eating and drinking, personal hygiene and handwriting. Up to now, the opinion of persons with intention tremor was rarely reported to this extent. The highlighted activities of daily life must be considered carefully in the design of future studies investigating the efficacy of therapy programs for tremor.

REFERENCES

Armutlu, K., Karabudak, R., & Nurlu, G. (2001). Physiotherapy approaches in the treatment of ataxic multiple sclerosis: A pilot study. *Neurorehabilitation and Neural Repair, 15* (3), 203-211.

Alusi, S. H., Glickman, S., Aziz, T. Z., & Bain, P. G. (1999). Tremor in multiple sclerosis [editorial]. *Journal of Neurology, Neurosurgery and Psychiatry, 66*(2), 131-134.

Alusi, S. H., Worthington, J., Glickman, S., & Bain, P. G. (2001). A study of tremor in multiple sclerosis. *Brain, 124*(Pt 4), 720-730.

Bain, P. G., Findley, L. J., Atchison, P., Behari, M., Vidailhet, M., Gresty, M., Rothwell, J. C., Thompson, P. D., & Marsden, C. D. (1993). Assessing tremor severity. *Journal of Neurology, Neurosurgery and Psychiatry, 56*(8), 868-873.

Bastian, A. J. (1997). Mechanisms of ataxia. *Physical Therapy, 77*(6), 672-675.

Beatty, W. W., & Goodkin, D. E. (1990). Screening for cognitive impairment in multiple sclerosis. An evaluation of the Mini-Mental State Examination. *Archives of Neurology, 47*(3), 297-301.

Dahlin-Webb, S. R. (1986). A weighted wrist cuff. *American Journal of Occupational Therapy, 40*(5), 363-364.

Deuschl, G., Bain, P., & Brin, M. (1998). Consensus statement of the Movement Disorder Society on Tremor. Ad Hoc Scientific Committee. *Movement Disorders, 13*(Suppl 3), 2-23.

Deuschl, G., Wenzelburger, R., Loffler, K., Raethjen, J., & Stolze, H. (2000). Essential tremor and cerebellar dysfunction: Clinical and kinematic analysis of intention tremor. *Brain, 123*(Pt 8), 1568-1580.

Ebers, G. C., Sadovnick, A.D. (1998). Chapter 2: Epidemiology. In D. W. Paty, & Ebers, G.C. (Ed.), *Multiple Sclerosis* (pp. 5-28). Philadelphia: F.A. Davis Company.

Feys, P., Duportail, M., Kos, D., Van Asch, P., & Ketelaer, P. (2002). Validity of the TEMPA for the measurement of upper limb function in multiple sclerosis. *Clinical Rehabilitation, 16*(2), 166-173.

Feys, P., Helsen, W., Liu, X., Loontjens, V., Lavrysen, A., Nuttin, B., & Ketelaer, P. (in press). Effect of visual information on step-tracking movements in patients with intention tremor due to multiple sclerosis. *Multiple Sclerosis.*

Feys, P., Helsen, W. F., Lavrysen, A., Nuttin, B., & Ketelaer, P. (2003a). Intention tremor during manual aiming: A study of eye and hand movements. *Multiple Sclerosis, 9*(1), 44-54.

Feys, P., Romberg, A., Ruutiainen, J., Davies-Smith, A., Jones, R., Avizzano, C. A., Bergamasco, M., & Ketelaer, P. (2001). Assistive technology to improve PC interaction for people with intention tremor. *Journal of Rehabilitation, Research and Development, 38*(2), 235-243.

Feys, P. G., Davies-Smith, A., Jones, R., Romberg, A., Ruutiainen, J., Helsen, W. F., & Ketelaer, P. (2003b). Intention tremor rated according to different finger-to-nose test protocols: A survey. *Archives of Physical Medicine and Rehabilitation, 84*(1), 79-82.

Folstein, M. F., Folstein, S. E., & McHugh, P. R. (1975). "Mini-mental state": A practical method for grading the cognitive state of patients for the clinician. *Journal of Psychiatry Research, 12*(3), 189-198.

Gillen, G. (2000). Improving activities of daily living performance in an adult with ataxia. *American Journal of Occupational Therapy, 54*(1), 89-96.

Granger, C. V., Cotter, A. C., Hamilton, B. B., Fiedler, R. C., & Hens, M. M. (1990). Functional assessment scales: A study of persons with multiple sclerosis. *Archives of Physical Medicine and Rehabilitation, 71*(11), 870-875.

Hooper, J., Taylor, R., Pentland, B., & Whittle, I. R. (1998). Rater reliability of Fahn's tremor rating scale in patients with multiple sclerosis. *Archives of Physical Medicine and Rehabilitation, 79*(9), 1076-1079.

Jones, L., Lewis, Y., Harrisson, J., & Wiles, C. M. (1996). The effectiveness of occupational therapy and physiotherapy in multiple sclerosis patients with ataxia of the upper limb and trunk. *Clinical Rehabilitation, 10,* 277-282.

Kesselring, J., & Thompson, A. J. (1997). Spasticity, ataxia and fatigue in multiple sclerosis. *Baillieres Clinical Neurology, 6*(3), 429-445.

Ketola, T. (1995). Psychology of ataxia in patients with MS. In P. Ketelaer & J. Ruutiainen (Eds.), *Ataxia* (pp. 53-56). Genova: A.I.S.M.

Kraft, G. H. (1998). Rehabilitation principles for patients with multiple sclerosis. *Journal of Spinal Cord Medicine, 21*(2), 117-120.

Kurtzke, J. F. (1983). Rating neurologic impairment in multiple sclerosis: An expanded disability status scale (EDSS). *Neurology, 33*(11), 1444-1452.

Langdon, D. W., & Thompson, A. J. (1999). Multiple sclerosis: A preliminary study of selected variables affecting rehabilitation outcome. *Multiple Sclerosis, 5*(2), 94-100.

Linacre, J. M., Heinemann, A. W., Wright, B. D., Granger, C. V., & Hamilton, B. B. (1994). The structure and stability of the Functional Independence Measure. *Archives of Physical Medicine and Rehabilitation, 75*(2), 127-132.

Liu, X., Miall, C., Aziz, T. Z., Palace, J. A., Haggard, P. N., & Stein, J. F. (1997). Analysis of action tremor and impaired control of movement velocity in multiple sclerosis during visually guided wrist-tracking tasks. *Movement Disorders, 12*(6), 992-999.

Matsumoto, J., Morrow, D., Kaufman, K., Davis, D., Ahlskog, J. E., Walker, A., Sneve, D., Noseworthy, J., & Rodriguez, M. (2001). Surgical therapy for tremor in multiple sclerosis: An evaluation of outcome measures. *Neurology, 57*(10), 1876-1882.

Morrice, B. L., Becker, W. J., Hoffer, J. A., & Lee, R. G. (1990). Manual tracking performance in patients with cerebellar incoordination: Effects of mechanical loading. *Canadian Journal of the Neurological Sciences, 17*(3), 275-285.

Nakamura, R., Kamakura, K., Tadano, Y., Hosoda, Y., Nagata, N., Tsuchiya, K., Iwata, M., & Shibasaki, H. (1993). MR imaging findings of tremors associated with lesions in cerebellar outflow tracts: Report of two cases. *Movement Disorders, 8*(2), 209-212.

Niranjan, A., Kondziolka, D., Baser, S., Heyman, R., & Lunsford, L. D. (2000). Functional outcomes after gamma knife thalamotomy for essential tremor and MS-related tremor. *Neurology, 55*(3), 443-446.

Ruutiainen, J. (1997). Assessment and treatment of ataxia in multiple sclerosis. In P. Ketelaer, M. Prosiegel, M. Battaglia, & U. Messmer (Eds.), *A Problem-oriented Approach to Multiple Sclerosis* (pp. 227-235). Leuven: Amersfoort.

Schenk, T., Walther, E. U., & Mai, N. (2000). Closed- and open-loop handwriting performance in patients with multiple sclerosis. *European Journal of Neurology, 7*(3), 269-279.

Sharrack, B., Hughes, R. A., Soudain, S., & Dunn, G. (1999). The psychometric properties of clinical rating scales used in multiple sclerosis. *Brain, 122*(Pt 1), 141-159.

Sheikh, K., Smith, D. S., Meade, T. W., Goldenberg, E., Brennan, P. J., & Kinsella, G. (1979). Repeatability and validity of a modified activities of daily living (ADL) index in studies of chronic disability. *International Rehabilitation Medicine, 1*(2), 51-58.

Weinshenker, B. G., Issa, M., & Baskerville, J. (1996). Long-term and short-term outcome of multiple sclerosis. A 3-year follow-up study. *Archives of Neurology, 53*, 353-358.

Wellingham-Jones, P. (1991). Characteristics of handwriting of subjects with multiple sclerosis. *Perceptual Motor Skills, 73*(3 Pt 1), 867-879.

Yuen, H. K. (1993). Self-feeding system for an adult with head injury and severe ataxia. *American Journal of Occupational Therapy, 47*(5), 444-451.

Developing and Implementing Lifestyle Management Programs[©] with People with Multiple Sclerosis

Christa Roessler, AccOT BAppSc(OT)Cumb
Jenny Barling, AccOT BAppSc(OT)Cumb
Megan Dephoff, AccOT BHlthSc(OT)
Terri Johnson, OTR BSc(OT)
Susan Sweeney, BAppSc(OT)Cumb

SUMMARY. This paper describes the development and use of Lifestyle Management Programs [©](LMPs) by occupational therapists at the Multiple Sclerosis Society of New South Wales, Australia. A case study is used to demonstrate how the program is applied in an individual situation. LMPs are used with people with MS, or their support people, to enable management of the impact of fluctuating and interactive physical, sensory and cognitive symptoms. LMPs are flexible and adaptable systems, allowing integration of information and strategies for managing symptoms. LMPs assist clients to sustain meaningful activities and life roles. Subjective client feedback supports the effectiveness of the pro-

---

Christa Roessler, Jenny Barling, Megan Dephoff, Terri Johnson, and Susan Sweeney are all affiliated with Rehabilitation Services-Occupational Therapy, MS Society of NSW, PO Box 210, Lidcombe, Australia (E-mail: ot@msnsw.org.au).

[Haworth co-indexing entry note]: "Developing and Implementing Lifestyle Management Programs[©] with People with Multiple Sclerosis." Roessler, Christa et al. Co-published simultaneously in *Occupational Therapy in Health Care* (The Haworth Press,) Vol. 17, No. 3/4, 2003, pp. 97-114; and: *Occupational Therapy Practice and Research with Persons with Multiple Sclerosis* (ed: Marcia Finlayson) The Haworth Press, Inc., 2003, pp. 97-114. Single or multiple copies of this article are available for a fee from The Haworth Document Delivery Service [1-800-HAWORTH, 9:00 a.m. - 5:00 p.m. (EST). E-mail address: docdelivery@haworthpress.com].

10.1300/J003v17n03_07

grams in meeting specific individual goals. Formal outcome measures are being explored. *[Article copies available for a fee from The Haworth Document Delivery Service: 1-800-HAWORTH. E-mail address: <docdelivery@haworthpress. com> Website: <http://www.HaworthPress.com> © 2003 by The Haworth Press, Inc. All rights reserved.]*

KEYWORDS. Lifestyle management, multiple sclerosis, rehabilitation, symptom management, cognition, memory, fatigue, management strategies

INTRODUCTION

Maintaining a fulfilling lifestyle, including work, family and leisure time, presents a daily challenge to everyone. People living with multiple sclerosis (MS) face an additional challenge in that they commonly experience symptoms that fluctuate and interact to have a significant impact on lifestyle and life-role satisfaction. Physical symptoms characterizing MS include weakness, sensation changes, bladder and bowel dysfunction, visual changes, tremor and balance problems. Other less obvious symptoms of MS, though no less common, include fatigue and cognitive changes. These are often referred to as 'silent' symptoms as they are more difficult to recognize and detect (Bagert, Complair & Bourdette, 2002; Johnson & Blumhardt, 2002; Lisak, 2001). The functional impact of all these symptoms often adversely affects the individual, family and support networks. Planning and organizing daily activities can become more difficult as the person must incorporate symptom management with the completion of daily tasks. If this challenge is further complicated by some degree of cognitive impairment and/or fatigue, the individual may feel overwhelmed with all they need to do and remember during the course of their daily lives.

How does the person with MS overcome the obstacles they face in carrying out life's daily tasks and roles? As a health professional, how is it possible to enable a person with MS to manage interactive, fluctuating, and diverse symptoms to achieve their occupational potential? These are the questions that led the occupational therapists at the MS Society of New South Wales (NSW), Australia to investigate available evidence and resources, to determine the best way to enable people to manage daily life despite unpredictable and variable symptoms. This process of inquiry eventuated in the development of the Lifestyle Management Program© (2001). The Lifestyle Management Program© (LMP) is a unique concept that facilitates the practical application, adaptation and integration of information and management strategies into daily life for individuals, their families, and support networks.

Underpinning the development of the LMP is the Occupational Performance Model (Australia) [OPM(A)]. This approach focuses on "addressing client's occupational needs" (Chapparo & Ranka, 1997, p. 52). The OPM(A) provides a framework that encompasses all contributing factors to a person's occupational roles. In providing 'programs,' occupational therapists assist clients to adapt to fundamental changes in components of occupational performance. This approach ensures that "all aspects of human function that contribute to occupational performance are considered" (Chapparo & Ranka, p. 52).

An individual LMP is a physical compilation of ideas, worksheets, information, and suggestions that usually takes the form of a calendar, notebook, or organizer. An individual LMP is coordinated by one health professional, but may include contributions from other team members, service providers, family, and carers. The individual program is created with and named by the client to reflect his or her lifestyle and occupations. The label of 'program' was deliberately chosen so there were no pre-conceived ideas about what a program may entail. That is, the concept is broader than just a diary or organizer.

An individual LMP is made up of a series of templates, flow charts, checklists, or other resources a person needs, to create a solution-oriented and practical record of daily life. It is a working system that allows the individual to prospectively plan, check, and communicate their needs; perform in the moment, and also have a retrospective record of achievement. For example, a program kept in a folder may contain a sheet of fitness exercises, a phone list, an activity schedule, a checklist to assist with planning a bus trip, or a list of fatigue management strategies. However, programs can take other forms, such as an individualized wall calendar, message board, or pager system. Essentially, an individual LMP is created and adapted to include whatever the client needs to fulfill their occupational potential.

Background

The MS Society of NSW uses a client-centered, needs-based approach to service provision to nearly 4000 registered clients across the state of NSW, Australia. Amongst other specialized services, clients have access to the rehabilitation team including occupational therapy, physiotherapy, clinical psychology, and neuropsychology. This team provides comprehensive assessment, intervention, education, and consultation to people with MS, their families and carers, as well as service providers, and community- and hospital-based health professionals.

The occupational therapists at the MS Society of NSW, provide current, evidence-based management strategies and information to clients who identify difficulty managing activities and life roles due to the impact of MS symptoms. These strategies and information are drawn from comprehensive education packages developed by the occupational therapists to assist in managing commonly identified symptoms, including fatigue and memory problems. The packages, which are reviewed annually, are based on current literature outlining best practice and contain specific information, assessment and management strategies. Initially, the information in these packages formed the basis for specific therapy with individuals. However, over a period of time it became apparent that despite comprehensive assessment and intervention using the education packages, clients were returning to occupational therapy with similar difficulties to those initially identified. While many clients were able to articulate information and strategies previously learned in therapy sessions and from handouts in regard to management of particular MS symptoms, actual application to daily life proved to be more challenging. Clients reported feeling overwhelmed with the large range of information received from various sources about individual topics related to MS. For example, information from a nurse about immunotherapy and continence management; information from a psychologist about emotional well-being; information from a neurologist, the Internet, other support people and so on. In addition, many described difficulty integrating and balancing management strategies for a range of fluctuating and interactive symptoms, within the context of home and community life.

LMPs for individuals are compiled into a format that has application and meaning for the person and their lifestyle. The LMP is the result of simplifying, coordinating, and integrating evidence-based strategies and information drawn from literature and practice. As part of the continuous review process to identify and meet client needs, the occupational therapists have established that similar strategies can be used to manage different symptoms. For example, a weekly schedule can be used to pace activities (fatigue management), and can also be used to plan and remember tasks (memory management).

PROGRAM DEVELOPMENT
AND IMPLEMENTATION FOR INDIVIDUALS

In understanding the overall concept of the LMP and how they are developed for individuals, clinicians need an understanding and appreciation of the range of MS symptoms and the functional effects these can have on occupational performance and lifestyle. It is also essential to have knowledge of current assessment and management strategies to be able to adapt these strategies to meet individual need and create the most applicable individual program. While it is not within the scope of this paper to address these issues in detail, a brief overview is necessary to provide a basis for the development of the LMP.

MS is the most common demyelinating disease of the central nervous system (Ben-Zacharia & Lublin, 2001) and predominantly a disease of young to middle-aged adults (Paty & Ebers, 1998). This is particularly significant when examining life roles usually associated with this stage of life–many people are embarking on careers or starting families. There is a strong risk of "lost work productivity" (Ben-Zacharia & Lublin, p. 801) that has the potential to be very costly to individuals and society.

A brief list of common symptoms has been noted in the introduction, along with the fact that symptoms are interactive in nature. This interaction is not commonly addressed in terms of management of symptoms. Client services staff at the MS Society of NSW frequently assesses people with MS who are experiencing a 'vicious circle' of symptoms where one or more symptoms interact with others, increasing impact on function. A common example of a client's experience demonstrates this symptom interaction well: A low-grade bladder infection may increase the core body temperature. In turn this may increase fatigue levels, which may cause the person to stop doing some activities. A lower level of activity may lead to deconditioning and increased weakness. Higher levels of fatigue may also affect the person's ability to concentrate, further affecting ability to take in information. Where the person has not been able to absorb information, memory problems may be further exacerbated. This example clearly highlights the breadth and often overwhelming 'picture' of difficulties MS may perpetuate.

In developing LMPs for individuals, the therapist working with a person with MS should be aware of the person's specific physical and sensory status, and the impact these symptoms have on their functional abilities. The format of an LMP will vary depending on an individual's ability to complete tasks including writing, reading specific size font, using a computer if required, turning pages, and lifting and carrying a folder, for example.

Fatigue

MS fatigue is experienced by about 75-95% of people with MS (Multiple Sclerosis Council for Clinical Practice Guidelines [MSCCPG], 1998). Fatigue is defined as a "subjective lack of physical energy and mental energy, that is perceived by the individual or caregiver to interfere with usual and desired activities" (MSCCPG, p. 2). It is associated with subjective feelings of tiredness, weakness and/or lack of energy after prolonged or excessive periods of either physical or mental activity (Merkelbach, Sittinger & Koenig, 2002). Further, it is defined as being distinct from sadness, although depression is closely linked with perceptions of fatigue. The experience of fatigue is regardless of the level of physical disability. Fatigue is reported as the single most common complaint (Lisak, 2001; MSCCPG, 1998; Schwid, Covington, Segal & Goodman, 2002; Taylor & Taylor, 1998) and has been implicated along with cognitive changes as the main cause of employment loss (Krupp & Rizvi, 2002; MSCCPG, 1998).

Assessment of fatigue by the occupational therapists at the MS Society of NSW entails a comprehensive initial interview and the completion of the Modified Fatigue Impact Scale. While this scale does not have any normative data, the occupational therapists find it helpful in a qualitative capacity as a basis for identifying and discussing key problem areas. It has also been identified as the 'best' tool based on the evidence compiled by the MS Council for Clinical Practice Guidelines (1998), although health professionals are exhorted to research its clinical utility further. Activity analysis, fatigue diaries, energy conservation, and education are also central to assessment and management of fatigue.

Cognition

Cognitive changes are relatively common among people with MS. Overall, between 43-65% (Rao et al., 1991) of people with MS experience cognitive changes in one or more of the following areas: Short-term memory, speed of information processing, attention, concentration, verbal fluency, visual-spatial abilities, and executive functioning (Bagert et al., 2002; Ben-Zacharia & Lublin, 2001; Britell, 1998). Executive functioning includes planning, organization, decision-making, reasoning, problem solving, initiation, and self-monitoring.

Previous studies have found that a significant number of people with MS with minimal physical difficulties experienced cognitive impairments severe enough to preclude employment, cause social isolation, and disrupt social functioning and other activities of daily living (Beatty, 1993; Beatty & Scott, 1993; Krupp & Rivzi, 2002; Rao et al., 1991). Cognitive impairment not only affects the person with MS to varying degrees, but can also have a significant impact on their families and carers' ability to practically and effectively provide assistance and support. An understanding of these difficulties is required not only by the individual but also by their support network to ensure consistency in planning, organizing, remembering, and executing programs (Nygård & Öhman, 2002).

Beatty (1993) notes that early detection of cognitive changes can promote understanding and direct rehabilitation efforts. This is especially pertinent when looking at implementing an LMP with a client, as their level of cognitive deficit will determine the success of the program, as well as equip the therapist with information to pitch the program at a level that the client is able to use. In assessing cognitive function, the Screening Examination for Cognitive Impairment (Beatty et al., 1995) is used as a routine and specific cognitive screening tool to assist in identifying and managing perceived problems, along with comprehensive interview, and self and family report.

The implementation and success of an individual LMP relies on the client having only mild to moderate cognitive impairment. Clients with any level of cognitive change need to have insight into their areas of difficulty, as well as an appreciation of the possibility to exercise some control over these difficulties through using management strategies. It follows that a good level of motivation combined with a goal-oriented approach will increase the chance of the client successfully utilizing a LMP.

In implementing an LMP, a supportive social environment will enhance motivation and success. It is therefore essential that family and carers are involved in the process of creating, implementing, and using the program. Where initiation of activity is an issue for an individual, it may be necessary to build in a reminder system such as an alarm or prompt from a family member.

It is well recognized that the experience of MS is very different for each person. This has implications for the development and implementation of an individual LMP. All symptoms of MS are individual and may fluctuate temporarily due to the time of day, stress, exacerbation, or increases in external heat or internal body temperature. To reflect this need for individual application, each person who identifies difficulties with the impact of symptoms on daily life has their LMP developed to reflect the wide range of activities, roles, and tasks that are involved in the person's lifestyle, balanced with symptom management. The adoption of a predictive and preventative approach teaches people not only how to use the program, but how to adapt and create new aspects as the need arises. Review and follow-up after the implementation of an LMP ensures that if a change of function or circumstance should occur, the program can be adjusted. The avenue to recontact the occupational therapists is open to all clients.

LITERATURE REVIEW

The LMP has developed in direct response to client need. As the program has evolved, the literature has been appraised to ascertain the existence of similar programs or concepts. No specialized programs were identified that focus on the integrated management of MS symptoms and reduction of the impact of symptoms on lifestyle. A review of the literature did reconfirm a number of cognitive rehabilitation and fatigue management strategies already being used. A brief overview of these will demonstrate how the LMP capitalizes on the successful principles of these strategies, and extends them to an individual's lifestyle.

The concept of the LMP does reflect similarities to research undertaken in the area of cognitive rehabilitation. Generally, cognitive rehabilitation strategies can be classed into restorative (remedial training of specific skills) and compensatory strategies (Britell, 1998; Tate, 1997). Examples of restorative strategies include mnemonics and other internal strategies like specific memory training, memory groups, medications, and vanishing cues. The use of external memory aids, which are compensatory strategies, is well documented and includes the use of personal organizers, calendars and tape recorders, memory notebooks and daily schedules (Bagert et al., 2002; Mateer & Sohlberg, 1988; Sohlberg & Raskin, 1996; Wilson, 2000). These aids aim to assist the person to organize and recall information by recording it in a systematic and easily accessible way. These authors suggest an individual and specific approach is crucial to the success of recommended strategies. A need for training in the use of external memory aids is also emphasized. Sullivan, Dehoux and Buchanan (1989) propose a cognitive intervention program specifically for people with MS that focuses on three areas: Structuring, scheduling, and recording. These intervention strategies can be successfully achieved through the use of calendars and notepads, and involves thorough assessment and training. Mateer and Sohlberg propose the use of memory notebooks with sections that address individually identified needs. Mateer and Sohlberg's study (along with a later study by Sullivan, Edgley and Dehoux, 1990) also note the essential aspect of 'prospective memory,' that is, planning ahead. This aspect of memory is often not addressed in research of memory difficulties where the focus is predominantly on recall of learned information.

Cognitive rehabilitation strategies have been implemented with varying degrees of success, predominantly with people with traumatic brain injuries, where there is the possibility of some cognitive improvement (Mateer & Sohlberg, 1988; Wilson, 2000). Published studies yielded some benefit to the participants; however, most acknowledged a significant limitation being the questionable application of learned skills to more generalized settings outside the rehabilitation environment.

Specific memory training can be beneficial when there is the possibility of improvement in memory and cognitive function. However, as cognitive problems in MS do not tend to improve over time due to nerve damage, the documented restorative memory rehabilitation strategies are not generally appropriate for people with MS. Literature suggests that compensatory strategies and environmental modifications are more likely to provide lasting benefits than direct retraining of specific skills (Bagert et al., 2002; Sohlberg & Raskin, 1996).

Nygård and Öhman (2002) recorded the personal experiences of a group of people with Alzheimer's Disease. This study revealed the successful strategies employed by the subjects to manage daily life, including written notes and diaries, checklists and timers and the use of habits and routines. Immediate action, reversing and repeating steps were also noted as common strategies. However, for people with MS where fatigue is also a common complaint, such strategies could contribute to unnecessary energy expenditure and forgoing essential rest breaks. People with MS require strategies that avoid repetition and facilitate planning.

There are a number of resources available in the literature outlining rehabilitation strategies for fatigue management. In 1998, the MS Council for Clinical Practice Guidelines (MSCCPG) published a comprehensive guide, which draws together current understanding and practice in multidisciplinary management of MS fatigue. This guide was developed to address the gap in empirical evidence as to the efficacy of commonly used treatments and interventions. The guide includes an algorithm for eliminating potentially contributing factors such as depression, poor diet, and sleep disturbance, as well as managing the effects of MS fatigue. Strategies include medication, fitness, education, heat reduction, and energy conservation.

There is evidence available in the literature that supports particular facets of overall fatigue management. For example, one aspect of fatigue management is using energy conservation principles as noted in the MSCCPG. Mathiowetz, Matuska and Murphy (2001) undertook an energy conservation program specifically with a group of people with MS and found benefit in immediate and short-term outcomes. This course was based on a program developed by Packer, Brink and Sauriol (1995) called "Managing Fatigue." The worksheets and strategies outlined in this program serve as a concrete reference for participants. However, this program, as with others, only addresses this one facet of MS symptom management.

There is some acknowledgement in the literature of the interaction of symptoms (Krupp & Christodoulou, 2001; Schwid et al., 2002). This acknowledgement supports the need for multidisciplinary rehabilitation strategies to assist people to manage their lifestyles in a sustainable and satisfactory way (Freeman, Hobart & Thompson, 1996; Johnson & Blumhardt, 2002; Thompson, 2002). Specific reference to the concept of 'lifestyle management' does not arise in the literature apart from some references to 'healthy lifestyles' and lifestyle modification for people with conditions such as diabetes or heart disease (Clark & Hampson, 2001). However, the way in which these lifestyle modification programs are individualized and client-centered demonstrates a need for practical application that is addressed in the way LMPs are developed for individuals.

In summary, the literature supports using a number of rehabilitative strategies to enable the person with MS experiencing difficulties to compensate for the impact of MS symptoms. These compensatory strategies facilitate function, occupational performance, and quality of life (Ben-Zacharia & Lublin, 2001; Johnson & Blumhardt, 2002; Langdon & Thompson, 1999). However, as demonstrated, the literature presents little information to health professionals or people with MS in regard to combining a range of strategies in a meaningful and individual way.

CASE EXAMPLE: SUE

Sue is 32 years old, married and has three young children, ages 7, 5, and 3 years. Sue defines her primary roles as homemaker and mother. Sue previously worked as an administrative assistant, however, stopped working when she had her first child. Her husband Ed works long hours as a real-estate agent. Sue was diagnosed with MS three months ago.

Sue's physical status fluctuates. She has occasional problems with balance, blurred vision, and sensation changes in her hands. These symptoms are transient and do not generally cause any difficulty with occupational performance. She experiences urinary incontinence and manages this by self-catheterizing three times a day. Severe fatigue is identified as Sue's primary problem. She is constantly tired, and has difficulty completing all the tasks that her busy lifestyle usually involves. Sue says planning and organizing for herself and her family is becoming more difficult and she is forgetting things. She has tried writing reminders on pieces of paper and in a notebook; however, she has found this method to be unsatisfactory. Neuropsychological testing showed only minor changes with speed of information processing.

Both Sue and Ed are having difficulty adjusting to Sue's diagnosis. Sue says she is beginning to feel anxious and depressed by all the recent changes and feels that she is 'losing control.' Her emotional status contributes to the difficulties she is experiencing. At a time when Sue needs more support, the family feels overwhelmed by Sue's reactions and their added responsibilities completing extra tasks that she is usually able to do, such as shopping, cooking, housekeeping, and child-care.

Sue has identified the following goals: To complete more household tasks including shopping, light cleaning and laundry, and to cook meals at home five nights per week. She would also like to spend more time with her youngest child each day and time after school with the two older children. Sue wants to be able to plan her routine and remember the children's schedules and appointments, and generally be able to manage her memory difficulties more efficiently and consistently.

Sue was referred for a 'team assessment' at the MS Society of NSW. Specifically, for occupational therapy assessment and management of symptoms that were affecting her ability to carry out her roles to her satisfaction. As Sue was newly-diagnosed, she and her family knew little about MS, symptoms, and management. One outcome of occupational therapy intervention was the development of an individual LMP that enabled Sue to integrate, monitor, and apply the strategies and information recommended, not just by occupational therapy, but also by other health professionals.

Sue and Ed were both very involved in setting goals and planning Sue's program together with the occupational therapist. An outline of some of the templates in Sue's program are listed and figures showing parts of the actual pages are included. The physical format of Sue's program was an A4 (21cm × 29.7cm) size 3-ring binder with section dividers.

Templates

Title Page. Sue's children watched a television program in which one of the characters had a "Handy Dandy Watch" he referred to frequently. Sue named her notebook "Handy Dandy Notebook" so her children could relate to it more easily.

My Week at Home. This is a list of all the possible activities Sue might need to complete in any week. Sue used this template as a prompt to remember what activities she needed to schedule.

Weekly Schedule. Sue's weekly schedule had no set time divisions, as she preferred to schedule the order of activities in her day around set events such as meals. She, Ed, and the children spent time together every Sunday evening planning their schedules for the upcoming week.

Meal Planning. This template allows meals and required ingredients to be listed and can generate a shopping list. Sue sat down each Sunday night after dinner with her family to plan meals for the week. Each person in the family chose the meal for one night. This became a family activity the children looked forward to each week (see Figure 1).

Ed's "Honey Do" List. Sue used this template to record jobs she wanted Ed to complete. Ed looked in Sue's notebook to check the list once a week.

Sue's "Honey Do" List. Ed used this template to record jobs he wanted Sue to complete. Sue checked the list twice a day to establish what needed to be done, and then to check what tasks remained (see Figure 2).

Telephone and Visitor's Messages. Sue and Ed frequently argued because Sue forgot to pass on important messages. Sue agreed to write down all messages for Ed on this template, and Ed agreed it would be his responsibility to check Sue's notebook for messages each evening.

Fun Things. Sue tended to work at completing all her "jobs" and leave no time for leisure. This template helped remind Sue that a balanced lifestyle is important for maintaining health. The template lists

FIGURE 1. Meal Planning Template

Meal Planning		
Day	**Meal**	**Shopping List**
Mon	Spaghetti bolognaise	Mince, tin tomato, cheese . . .
Tues	Vegetable stir-fry	Capsicum, snow peas, onion. . . . . .
Wed	Fish & chips & salad	Frozen fish, frozen chips, lettuce, tomato. . .
Thurs. . .	Dinner out	------------------

FIGURE 2. "Honey-Do List" Template

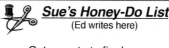

Sue's Honey-Do List
(Ed writes here)

- Get a quote to fix door
- Mend button on my grey pants
- Organize receipts for tax return
- Buy sports socks for David

activities that Sue has identified as 'fun' and which she can add to her weekly schedule.

Remembering Names. Sue took Polaroid photos of people whose names she had difficulty remembering and put the photos, along with the person's name, on this template for reference.

Project Plans. Sue used this template to outline major projects to be completed in more manageable steps (see Figure 3).

FIGURE 3. "Project Plans" Template

Project Plans

Project: ____   *Clean out linen closet* _____

Steps to complete task:

- ⁻ label boxes into categories eg. towels, sheets
- ⁻ sort everything into labelled boxes
- - clean shelves
- ⁻ put everything back

Things I need to organize:

- - get 6 empty boxes and label
- - put cleaning things together–bucket, cloth
- - plastic bags for throw–away

Outcome of project: closet sorted and cleaned, easy to see and find everything
---

Sue also had a business card holder in the program and plastic sleeves that allowed her to carry items such medication prescriptions and bills. There was a section for 'School' where all the information for her children's schedules was stored and a 'Health' section that contained her exercise program prescribed by a physiotherapist, a medication schedule, rest schedule, and questions she wanted to remember to ask her neurologist. Sue kept her program on the kitchen bench next to the telephone so that she did not have to 'remember' where it was. Meal breaks were used as prompts to check the program three times a day.

On review of the program, Sue reported that she met her goal of resuming and completing many of her daily tasks and roles. She felt she had more control over the impact of the disease with its unpredictable and fluctuating nature. Following Sue's orientation to the LMP, she reported she was very committed to using her notebook and carried it with her at all times when she went out. Her husband and children also became involved in the program. For example, Sue's children would often remind her to check her 'Handy Dandy Notebook.' The message page eliminated many arguments between Sue and Ed, leading to reduced household stress. Scheduling activities and sticking to her rest program helped Sue manage her fatigue very well, which meant she was able to meet all her goals related to household tasks and child care.

CONCLUSION

As the concept of LMPs developed and evolved, specific outcome measures began to be explored. Measures of change in specific behaviours or symptoms have traditionally been used to show the outcome of rehabilitation. However, for many people with MS, where there is permanent nerve damage, improvement of a specific symptom may not be a reasonable expectation. Given the nature of MS, adaptation to fluctuating function may be a more useful outcome. Therefore, measures of change in the ability to participate in and complete tasks that are important to the individual may be more reasonable and reflective of the benefits of intervention.

As the subject matter of LMPs is so diverse and individual, a measure addressing the impact the program has on lifestyle needs to be the key focus. To this end, goal attainment scales (GAS) are being investigated as the most appropriate measure to record and demonstrate individual change. GAS "evaluates program effectiveness by measuring the extent to which individual client goals are achieved in a specified time frame" (Cox & Amsters, 2002, p. 256). GAS acknowledges the individual nature of clients' issues and the multidisciplinary focus of the team (Cox & Amsters, 2002; Forbes, 1998) and has been used with a variety of client populations.

Using GAS, realistic, relevant, and specific goals are formed collaboratively between the clinician and the client to measure change in the client's performance over time (Ottenbacher & Cusick, 1990). Goal setting is important for motivation and clear expectations when formulating an intervention program. Goals need to be "measurable, attainable, desirable and socially, functionally, and contextually relevant" (Malec, 1999, p. 254). These concepts complement LMPs, which aim to assist the individual to achieve their goals within their unique context.

Anecdotal feedback directly from clients has demonstrated that individual LMPs make a positive difference to people's lifestyles. Clients have reported an increased ability to complete more tasks throughout the day and week, without feeling as fatigued. Many also report an improvement in managing memory problems by having a record of important information kept together in one location. One reported outcome of program use has been a decrease in anxiety levels. Many clients have said that using the program decreases stress associated with trying to remember things and fearing forgetting important information or schedules. Clients have reported being able to more effectively manage and organize their daily activities by the use of an integrated record of information.

Families and carers of more severely cognitively impaired clients have provided positive feedback about the usefulness of the program for organization of multiple services, medications and routines, as well as a concrete record as evidence of accomplishments. As LMPs are client-focused intervention strategies, measuring the success of intervention is complemented by client report of the usefulness of the program in achieving goals.

NOTE

Information regarding Lifestyle Management Programs can be obtained from: Occupational Therapy, MS Society of NSW, PO Box 210, Lidcombe, Australia (E-mail: ot@msnsw.org.au). © 2001 Multiple Sclerosis Society of New South Wales, Australia

REFERENCES

Bagert, B., Camplair, P. & Bourdette, D. (2002). Cognitive dysfunction in multiple sclerosis: Natural history, pathophysiology and management. *CNS Drugs, 16(7)*, 445-455.

Beatty, W.W., Paul, R.H., Wilbanks, S.L., Hames, K.A., Blanco, C.R. & Goodkin, D.E. (1995). Identifying multiple sclerosis patients with mild or global cognitive impairment using the Screening Examination for Cognitive Impairment (SEFCI). *Neurology, 45*, 718-723.

Beatty, W.W. & Scott, J.G. (1993). Issues and developments in the neuropsychological assessment of patients with multiple sclerosis. *Journal of Neurological Rehabilitation, 7(3/4)*, 87-97.

Beatty, W.W. (1993). Cognitive and emotional disturbances in multiple sclerosis. *Neurologic Clinics, 11*(1), 189-204.

Ben-Zacharia, A.B. & Lublin, F.D. (2001). Palliative care in patients with multiple sclerosis. *Neurologic Clinics, 19*(4), 801-827.

Britell, C.W. (1998). MS and cognitive function. *Multiple Sclerosis Quarterly Report, 17(1)*, 1-5.

Chapparo, C. & Ranka, J. (eds.) (1997). *Occupational Performance Model (Australia) Monograph 1*. Sydney: Occupational Performance Network.

Clark, M. & Hampson, S.E. (2001). Implementing a psychological intervention to improve lifestyle self-management in patients with type 2 diabetes. *Patient Education and Counselling, 42* (8), 247-256.

Cox, R. & Amsters, D. (2002). Goal attainment scaling: An effective outcome measure for rural and remote health services. *Australian Journal of Rural Health, 10* (5), 256-261.

Forbes, D. (1998). Goal attainment scaling: A responsive measure of client outcome. *Journal of Gerontological Nursing, 24*(12), 34-40.

Freeman, J.A., Hobart, J.C. & Thompson, A.J. (1996). Outcomes-based research in neurorehabilitation: The need for multidisciplinary team involvement. *Disability and Rehabilitation, 18*(2), 106-110.

Johnson, K.P. & Blumhardt, L.D. (2002). Practical issues in the management of multiple sclerosis: Introduction. *Neurology, 58(4)*, S1-2.

Krupp, L.B. & Christodoulou, C. (2001). Fatigue in multiple sclerosis. *Current Neurology and Neuroscience Reports, 1*, 294-298.

Krupp, L.B. & Rizvi, S.A. (2002). Symptomatic therapy for underrecognized manifestations of multiple sclerosis. *Neurology, 58*(4), S32-39.

Langdon, D.W. & Thompson, A.J. (1999). Multiple sclerosis: A preliminary study of selected variables affecting rehabilitation outcome. *Multiple Sclerosis, 5* (2), 94-100.

Lisak, D. (2001). Overview of symptomatic management of multiple sclerosis. *Journal of Neuroscience Nursing, 33(5)*, 224-230.

Malec, J. (1999). Goal attainment scaling in rehabilitation. *Neuropsychological Rehabilitation, 9*(3/4), 253-275.

Mateer, C.A. & Sohlberg, M.M. (1988). A paradigm shift in memory rehabilitation. In H. Whitaker (Ed.). *Neuropsychological Studies of Non-focal Brain Damage* (pp. 202-225). Springer Verlag.

Mathiowetz, V., Matuska, K.M. & Murphy, M.E. (2001). Efficacy of an energy conservation course for persons with multiple sclerosis. *Archives of Physical Medicine and Rehabilitation, 82(4)*, 449-456.

Merkelbach, S., Sittinger, H. & Koenig, J. (2002). Is there a differential impact of fatigue and physical disability on quality of life in multiple sclerosis? *The Journal of Nervous and Mental Disease, 190*(6), 388-393.

Multiple Sclerosis Council for Clinical Practice Guidelines [MSCCPG] (1998). *Fatigue and Multiple Sclerosis: Evidence Based Management Strategies for Fatigue in Multiple Sclerosis*. Washington, DC: Paralysed Veterans of America.

Nygård, L. & Öhman, A. (2002). Managing changes in everyday occupations: The experience of persons with Alzheimer's Disease. *Occupational Therapy Journal of Research, 22*(2), 70-81.

Ottenbacher, K.J. & Cusick, A. (1990). Goal attainment scaling as a method of clinical service evaluation. *The American Journal of Occupational Therapy, 44*, 519-525.

Packer, T.L., Brink, N. & Sauriol, A. (1995) *Managing Fatigue: A Six-week Course for Energy Conservation*. Tucson, AZ: Therapy Skill Builders.

Paty, D.W. & Ebers, G.C. (1998). *Multiple Sclerosis*. Philadelphia, PA: F.A. Davis Company.

Rao, S.M., Leo, G.J., Ellington, L., Nauertz, T., Bernardin, L. & Unverzagt, F. (1991) Cognitive dysfunction in multiple sclerosis II: Impact on employment and social functioning. *Neurology, 41* (5), 692-696.

Schwid, S.R., Covington, M., Segal, B.M. & Goodman, A.D. (2002). Fatigue in multiple sclerosis: Current understanding and future directions. *Journal of Rehabilitation Research and Development, 39(2)*, 211-224.

Sohlberg, M.M. & Raskin, S.A. (1996). Principles of generalization applied to attention and memory interventions. *Journal of Head Trauma Rehabilitation, 11*(2), 65-78.

Sullivan, M.J.L., Dehoux, E. & Buchanan, D.C. (1989). An approach to cognitive rehabilitation in multiple sclerosis. *Canadian Journal of Rehabilitation, 3*(2), 77-85.

Sullivan, M.J.L., Edgley, K. & Dehoux, E. (1990). A survey of multiple sclerosis. Part 1: Perceived cognitive problems and compensatory strategy use. *Canadian Journal of Rehabilitation, 4*(2), 99-105.

Tate, R.L. (1997). Subject review–Beyond one-bun, two-shoe: Recent advances in psychological rehabilitation of memory disorders acquired after brain injury. *Brain Injury, 11*(12), 907-918.

Taylor, A. & Taylor, R.S. (1998). Neuropsychologic aspects of multiple sclerosis. *Physical Medicine and Rehabilitation Clinics of North America, 9*(3), 643-657.

Thompson, A.J. (2002). Progress in neurorehabilitation in multiple sclerosis. *Current Opinion in Neurology, 15*(3), 267-270.

Wilson, B.A. (2000). Compensating for cognitive deficits following brain injury. *Neuropsychology Review, 10*(4), 233-243.

In Their Own Words:
Coping Processes Among Women
Aging with Multiple Sclerosis

Julie DalMonte, MS, OTR/L
Marcia Finlayson, PhD, OT(C), OTR/L
Christine Helfrich, PhD, OTR/L, FAOTA

SUMMARY. People with multiple sclerosis (MS) employ a variety of coping mechanisms throughout the process of managing their disease. This study describes the coping processes used by women aging with MS. Participants in the study included 23 women living in the Chicago area aged 55 years or older and diagnosed with MS for a minimum of 15

Julie DalMonte is Occupational Therapist, Lutheran Social Services of Illinois, Psychosocial Rehabilitation Program, 4840 W. Byron Street, Chicago, IL 60641.

Marcia Finlayson and Christine Helfrich are Assistant Professors, Department of Occupational Therapy, University of Illinois at Chicago, 1919 W. Taylor Street (Mail Code 811), Chicago, IL 60612-7250 (E-mail: marciaf@uic.edu).

This paper represents the thesis work of the first author.

Special thanks to the other individuals who contributed to conducting this study: Nadine Peacock, PhD (Co-Investigator), Toni Van Denend (Research Assistant), Edwin Loomis (Transcriptionist), and all of the participants.

The original study was funded through an award to Dr. Finlayson by the Campus Research Board at the University of Illinois at Chicago, July 2000-June 2001.

[Haworth co-indexing entry note]: "In Their Own Words: Coping Processes Among Women Aging with Multiple Sclerosis." DalMonte, Julie, Marcia Finlayson, and Christine Helfrich. Co-published simultaneously in *Occupational Therapy in Health Care* (The Haworth Press.) Vol. 17, No. 3/4, 2003, pp. 115-137; and: *Occupational Therapy Practice and Research with Persons with Multiple Sclerosis* (ed: Marcia Finlayson) The Haworth Press, Inc., 2003, pp. 115-137. Single or multiple copies of this article are available for a fee from The Haworth Document Delivery Service [1-800-HAWORTH, 9:00 a.m. - 5:00 p.m. (EST). E-mail address: docdelivery@haworthpress.com].

10.1300/J003v17n03_08

years. Data were gathered through in-depth semi-structured qualitative interviews. Findings suggest that participants who reported integrating MS into their lives, had confidence in their abilities to cope with stress, and had a positive outlook on life appeared to employ action-oriented strategies to cope with their disease. Findings from the study offer ideas and direction for occupational therapy interventions for women aging with multiple sclerosis. *[Article copies available for a fee from The Haworth Document Delivery Service: 1-800-HAWORTH. E-mail address: <docdelivery@haworth press.com> Website: <http://www.HaworthPress.com> © 2003 by The Haworth Press, Inc. All rights reserved.]*

KEYWORDS. Multiple sclerosis, mental health, coping, older adults, qualitative research

Multiple sclerosis (MS) is a chronic neurological disorder that is more common among women than men. It is characterized by inflammation of the central nervous system, sclerotic plaque formation, and axonal demyelination. Although pharmaceuticals are available that improve the course of the disease (e.g., Avonex ®, Betaseron® Copaxone®, and Rebif ®), there is currently no known cure. Nevertheless, having MS does not shorten life expectancy for the majority of individuals living with this disease (Weinshenker, 1995).

Major symptoms of MS include motoric weakness, fatigue, cognitive impairment, paresthesias, and problems in bladder, bowel, and sexual functioning (Aikens et al., 1999). In addition, mental health problems are often the consequence of the unpredictability and debilitating effects of the disease. Historically, much of the literature regarding mental health and MS has focused on problems such as depression and anxiety. In recent years some research has begun to address issues around coping and attitude, and how these factors influence the ability of people with MS to manage their disease and its consequences (Sullivan, Mikail, & Weinshenker, 1997; Fournier, de Ridder, & Bensing, 1999).

Aging poses unique challenges to people with MS as the disease can compound any decline in function associated with normal aging changes. Occupational therapists are particularly concerned with successful adaptation to disability stemming from chronic illness or age, and focus on maintaining or improving function of their clients through strategies that aid in coping, remediation or compensation (Christiansen & Baum, 1997). Because people aging with MS have been managing their disease for long periods of time and must simultaneously deal with the compounding influence of normal aging, their stories and perspectives may shed new light on successful as well as unsuccessful coping strategies relative to living with MS. Therefore, the purpose of this study was to understand and describe coping processes among women growing older with MS from their own perspectives.

LITERATURE REVIEW

Sinnakaruppan (2000) reports that coping and perception of coping are critical factors in dealing with chronic illnesses such as MS. Coping can be defined as "the strategies individuals use to minimize the negative impact of life stressors on their psychological well-being" (Sullivan et al., 1997 p. 250). A number of coping strategies have been identified in both the MS and non-MS literature and include, but are not exclusive to, denial (retreating from reality), suppression (avoiding the problem), focusing on the present, focusing on the positive, optimism, help-seeking, mapping (collecting information about the problem), and minimization (minimizing the importance of the problem) (Cohen & Lazarus, 1979).

In the literature on coping and MS, Sullivan et al. (1997) report suppression/avoidance, denial and focus on the present (i.e., taking one day at a time, thinking only of the challenges of what one has to do today) as strategies that are associated with low levels of depressive symptomology in people newly diagnosed with MS. Shontz (1975) suggests that suppression/avoidance and denial strategies may be considered positive if they inhibit the individual from becoming overwhelmed with the strain of illness (Shontz, 1975). In the early stages of illness, using suppression/avoidance and denial strategies may give the individual time to come to terms with frightening information about the new disability and its possible consequences, and to formulate alternative coping strategies (Lazarus, 1993; Shontz, 1975).

Other authors have argued that using the suppression/avoidance and denial strategies as primary coping mechanisms are connected with increased risk of depression in people who have MS or other chronic illnesses (Folkman, Chesney, Pollack, & Coates, 1993). Overall, the literature addressing suppression/avoidance and denial as a means of coping with MS has focused on young and middle aged adults. It is unknown the extent to which these strategies are used by older adults, and what the consequences of their use are for these individuals.

Positive focus and optimism have also been examined in studies of people with MS. Fournier et al. (1999) found that individuals with MS who responded to a mail-out survey and reported having optimistic expectations about the future and confidence in their abilities to cope with and manage stress appeared to maintain better mental health. The use of support groups, peer counselors, and the services of organizations such as the National Multiple Sclerosis Society to aid in coping with this disease are consistent with the strategies of help-seeking and mapping (collecting information about the problem) that have been described in the coping literature. Again, this literature does not address the use of these strategies among persons aging with multiple sclerosis.

In the coping literature concerning those people aging without MS, successful adaptation to increases in physical limitation has been associated with positive and optimistic moods in the very old (80+) non-MS population (Rubel, Reinsch, Tobis & Hurrell, 1994). In a study examining morale (confidence in self and satisfaction in life situation) and old age, Wenger, Davies and Shahtahmasebi (1995) found that in 534 people over 65 high morale was associated with continued mobility and feeling well, adequate income, spending minimal time alone, expecting care when ill from an informal care giver, and having a larger community support network. Downe-Wamboldt and Melanson (1998) found the most frequently used coping strategies employed by elderly people to manage the stress associated with rheumatoid arthritis were thinking positively about future outcomes and relying on one's own abilities and resources.

Literature concerning MS and coping, in addition to studies regarding normal aging and coping, support the need for closer examination of people aging with MS. As people with MS grow older, their symptoms may be compounded by the usual decline in function and increased risk of depression that accompanies aging (Bruce, Seeman, Merrill & Blazer, 1994). Subsequently, coping becomes crucial in the management of both emotional health and physical symptoms. Given the existing literature, the primary objective of this work was to develop an understanding of the coping strategies used by persons with MS. This paper is based on qualitative information gathered from in-depth semi-structured interviews. Throughout the paper, the words of the participants themselves will be directly quoted as often as possible. Some quantitative data will be used in order to provide basic descriptive information about the participants.

DESIGN AND METHODS

This study uses data collected from a broader study focusing on the health and service-related concerns of people aging with MS. Therefore, the methods of the original study are described below. The Institutional Review Board of the authors' university approved the study.

Participants

The voluntary participants of the original study consisted of 27 adults aging with MS. Inclusion criteria included having a birth date in or before 1947, having MS for at least 15 years, being able to carry on a conversation in English, and living in the Chicago area. People were excluded from the study if they felt they were physically or emotionally unable to tolerate the interview process (i.e., two 1½ to 2 hour interviews), and if they did not have a quiet and private location where the interview could be conducted.

Twenty-three females and four males participated in the original study. Because differences in coping strategies have been identified between men and women (O'Neill & Morrow, 2001; Malterud, Hollnagel & Witt, 2001), only the data from the women were included in this analysis. Table 1 provides basic demographic and health information about these 23 women. Though the study was open to people of any ethnic and/or racial background who met the criteria, all participants were Caucasian.

Procedures

Data for the study were collected from participants over a period of four months from August, 2001 to November, 2001. Participants for the study were recruited through the National Multiple Sclerosis Society (Greater Illinois Chapter). Recruitment through this organization consisted of advertisements about the study and a request for volunteers in the monthly newsletter sent to support group facilitators, who then distributed the advertisements to their members. Those support group members who were interested in participating contacted the study staff by phone to volunteer.

All potential participants were screened by telephone to meet eligibility requirements. At the time of the screening, eligible participants agreed upon a date and time for the formal consent process and the initial interview. Formal consent was acquired from participants at the start

TABLE 1. Demographic and Health Characteristics of Study Participants (N = 23)

Demographic Characteristics	Summary Statistics
Age in years	
Mean	61
Range	55-77
Marital status (counts)	
Married	15
Unmarried	8
Education	
12 or less years	7
More than 12 Years	15
Missing	1
Employment	
Retired	5
On disability	13
Homemaker	1
Working	3
Missing	1
Housing	
Single family home	16
Age integrated apartment	2
Condominium	2
Nursing home	2
Other accommodations	1
Multiple Sclerosis Characteristics	
Years of MS symptoms	
Mean	22
Range	15-39
Years since official diagnosis	
Mean	20
Range	6-39
Most common symptoms (counts)	
Fatigue	22
Loss of balance	20
Weakness	19
Pain	18
Spasticity	16
Currently taking medicine to relieve mental or emotional symptoms (count)	6
Self-reported mental health (count)	
Better now than 5 years ago	5
Same as 5 years ago	9
Worse now than 5 years ago	9

of the initial interview. Interviewers traveled to participants' homes or an agreed upon location to carry out the interviews. With the exception of two cases, interviews were conducted in the participant's home.

Data sources for the study included a guided, in-depth qualitative interview, and a set of standard rating scales and instruments commonly used in gerontological studies and/or studies of people with MS. Since fatigue was a factor for the participants, the interview process was divided into two sessions. The first session involved primarily the qualitative interview and basic demographic questions, and the second session consisted of follow-up questions from the initial interview, and the administration of the standardized instruments and scales. These two sessions were spaced between one and three weeks apart.

Instruments

Qualitative interviews were conducted by one of four trained interviewers in accordance with the interview guide. In all cases, participants gave permission for the interviews to be audiotaped and for the interviewer to take fieldnotes. The qualitative interview consisted of open-ended questions concerning participants' time use (e.g., describe what you do in a typical week), MS course and diagnosis (e.g., what led to your diagnosis of MS?), changes due to aging (e.g., have you noticed changes in yourself as you've gotten older?), concepts about health and aging (e.g., what does healthy mean to you?), and community service use and need (e.g., what services do you feel you need to stay healthy?). Coping strategies arose as a major point of discussion within the context of questions about managing MS, health and aging.

The quantitative interview using standardized instruments and scales consisted of the following measures: Multiple Sclerosis Quality of Life Inventory[1] and a modified version of the Older Americans Resources and Services Questionnaire (OARS). For the purpose of this paper, data from these sources were used for descriptive purposes only, and therefore they will not be discussed further. The data collected from the qualitative interview form the basis of this paper.

Analysis

The qualitative interviews were fully transcribed, converted to text files, and imported into a qualitative data analysis software program (ATLAS/ti) (Muhr, 1997). The coding scheme included investigator-generated constructs related to the purpose of the study (e.g. coping, social support, mental health, and service need), as well as respondent-generated themes that emerged from the narratives (e.g., burden, independence, advocate, and management strategies).

Three coders met at four to six week intervals throughout the coding process, during and after data collection, to compare coding decisions and discuss emerging themes to ensure dependability of the analysis process. The three coders created a list of qualitative codes and definitions based on the themes emerging from the data. Using these codes and definitions, these individuals completed an initial analysis of five of the interviews. The codes and definitions were then modified to better reflect the data. A second round of analysis was then done using the revised codes and definitions. After coding was completed, the retrieve feature of Atlas was used to extract codes and quotations reflecting major themes, and then these transcript excerpts were re-evaluated and recoded using codes that were more narrowly defined. The themes and sub-themes regarding coping used for this paper emerged from the qualitative interviews. Selected excerpts were chosen in order to illustrate major themes and definitions. Contrasting quotes were then chosen to explore the variability of the responses. For confidentiality, the names of the participants were changed.

RESULTS

From the qualitative interviews with the 23 women, two major themes emerged through the analysis of the data and are graphically depicted in Figure 1. Since one of the participants in the study exemplified the findings presented in this model, her case will be used to ground the presentation of the results. Quotes from other participants will be included to highlight or contrast significant concepts.

Carol's Story

Carol is a 59-year-old schoolteacher and mother of four grown children. She is a vibrant young-looking woman who uses no assistive devices for mobility. She is divorced and lives alone in a one-level house in a quiet suburb. Her children and grandchildren live nearby and she sees them often. Carol's parents are elderly and she shares care-taking responsibilities with her three siblings who live in the area. Her father is in poor health and her mother is unable to drive long distances. Carol is very involved in her church, and has a deep and profound faith in God.

FIGURE 1. Graphic Depiction of the Major Themes and Sub-themes Emerging from the Data Analysis

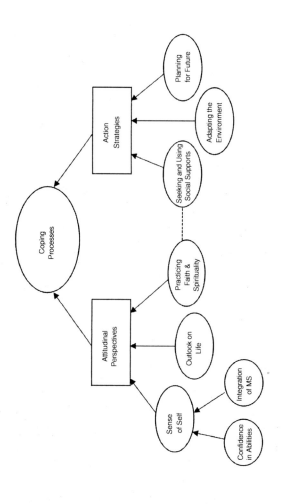

In addition to the many friends she has made through her involvement in MS support groups, Carol has several close friends without MS that she sees often. Carol walks slowly with a wide gait and experiences difficulty with balance. Currently, Carol has a slight case of nystagmus in her left eye and reports problems with focusing, especially when reading. She states that fatigue is a major issue for her, especially in the summer.

Carol was diagnosed with MS at age 43. Several years before her diagnosis, she noticed vision problems that disappeared almost as quickly as they came. The symptoms that led her to a MS diagnosis were numbness in her feet that gradually crept up to her waist, nystagmus, and balance problems. Carol describes her initial symptoms and the fear that accompanied them in this way:

> I woke up and the numbness had crept all the way up to my waist, and I thought, I think I'd better call the doctor because what if it continues going up? I was afraid it was going to affect my breathing you know and then if I couldn't breathe, I didn't want to die that way. I still don't want to die that way.

Throughout the course of her disease, Carol has had terrible episodes of nystagmus, sometimes making it impossible for her to see. Sudden attacks of severe vertigo also occur frequently. She compares her experience of having vertigo to a carnival ride:

> Carol: . . . now I know the neurologist did not understand me when I told him vertigo because he's thinking dizziness. This is so much worse than dizziness.

> Interviewer: Can you describe it?

> Carol: Well, I remember when I was a child. One time I went on this ride . . . you stand in this circle, this barrel and it spins around . . . and gradually the floor drops out and you are plastered to the wall . . . that's what it feels like . . . [and] the ride doesn't stop.

When Carol has these intense vertigo attacks, she is incapacitated. She must lie in bed and try not to move. She has a prescription drug that helps but she is sometimes unable to get it quickly. Fatigue is also a serious symptom that Carol experiences both during MS exacerbations (which seem to come every several years) and throughout remission periods. She states that she missed 9 weeks of school recently because of her fatigue.

While Carol's personal situation and experiences with MS are unique to her life, themes from her interview illustrate the major components of the model shown in Figure 1. Overall, the qualitative analysis revealed participants' coping processes as including two major themes: Attitudinal perspectives and active coping strategies.

Attitudinal Perspectives

Attitudinal perspectives are ways of thinking about oneself and the world that may either increase or decrease feelings of control, self-efficacy and mastery. Across the interviews, we found three factors that appeared to contribute to participants' attitudinal perspectives: Sense of self, outlook on life, and having faith and spirituality.

For Carol, she believes that the unpredictable course of her MS and her often debilitating symptoms played a hand in the recent disintegration of her marriage. After being married for 33 years, Carol's husband suddenly left her. Subsequently, Carol went through a deep depression. Her husband had taken care of many things when they were married, and she felt helpless without him. She was afraid of being alone, and of having an episode with her MS with no one there to help her:

> . . . when my husband left, that was really something that terrified me because it had been less than a year since I had an attack and I thought, what am I going to do? I mean, if I'm laying here and I can't move and nobody can get in the house and nobody even knows and everything, it was horrible, I utterly panicked.

Carol describes the end of her marriage as a "crisis point" and discusses it with some sadness and a bit of anger. Yet, her attitude towards the world now seems optimistic and hopeful. Through great heartache and struggle (Carol's MS continued to fluctuate between remission and severe attacks), a newfound confidence in her own abilities has emerged. She learned to do the things that her husband had always done. At first, she had no confidence in herself. Carol describes the change in her belief in her abilities:

> I was married for 33 years. And I'm also surprised that I can do as much as I can around the house. Like, I recaulked the bathtub last night. That's the sort of thing that my husband always took care of

because I couldn't do it. Whenever I would try to do any of those things that I couldn't do, I didn't do it quite right and so I learned no, he's right, you can't do it. And now I'm finding I can do a whole lot of this stuff that I had spent 33 years thinking I couldn't do.

Carol now seems to feel truly comfortable with herself and her autonomy. This crisis point in Carol's life ultimately had a beneficial effect on her. She discovered that she is able to take care of herself, manage her symptoms and be satisfied as a single woman:

I like my independence. In a sense I discovered it after I know it's been almost three years that he's gone. I really like living alone. I like that I can eat when I want to eat. I can eat what I want to eat and I can sleep when I want to sleep. I really like that. I didn't know that I would, you know.

Another way Carol copes with the symptoms of her MS is knowing and accepting her limitations and working around them. The integration of MS into herself and her life is an attitudinal perspective. However, both the confidence Carol has in her abilities and the acceptance she has of her limitations have led her to follow through with action strategies (Figure 1). She takes frequent naps and tries not to overexert herself by participating in too many activities, limiting her attendance at extracurricular activities at school because of her fatigue.

One of the ways that Carol and other participants in the study acknowledged their limitations was to plan for and work around the restrictions they experienced. A segment from an interview with Irene, a 57-year-old wife and mother of five grown children, illustrates this point:

[I] walk with two canes at home. Every floor has canes and walkers. It's like a hospital in there. But I'm doing it. The house, it's a bi-level . . . Acceptance. You have to be able to accept it.

But accepting limitations did not come easily for Carol, or for many of the other participants in the study. Gale, a 58-year-old married mother of two grown boys and a retired school counselor, describes how she denied having MS to herself and others for many years after her diagnosis:

For the early parts it (the MS) was mild and not really too noticeable and so, uh, it took me quite a while to kind of deal with it. I

think I was in denial for a long time . . . I would just make excuses
. . . oh I've got a bad knee or whatever, you know . . . [But then]
certain problems were sort of hanging around and it became obvious that they weren't going to go away . . . I never even called the
MS Society. I don't know, it was probably just a part of that denial
thing . . . as long as I didn't call, I didn't have to have it.

Though Carol has successfully integrated MS into herself and her
life, she still sometimes uses denial as a coping mechanism when she is
experiencing a remission:

I appreciate it. I mean I really do appreciate the fact that I am between exacerbations and I relish it . . . It makes it easier to deny
that it's ever going to hit me again because it feels normal. What
does it feel like? It's hard for me to say what it feels like. I just feel
happy.

For Carol, using both integration and denial at specific times throughout her disease course has helped her achieve independence in managing her MS. The ability of participants to integrate or not integrate MS
into their lives appeared to be related to the way they viewed themselves, the world around them, and their overall outlook on life. For
some participants, there was a perspective about life in general that was
present before MS. For others, the experience of living with MS has
reframed the way they view the world. Carol was faced with two traumatic life events at the same time, the end of her marriage and the progression of her disease. She can find the good in both now. Carol offers
insight into how MS has changed the way she looks at life:

I think it's helped me to take a solid look at what's truly important
in my life and life in general, and to put things in perspective and to
appreciate each day because I don't know.

Many participants described their positive attitudes as helping them
cope with life's stressors. For some, attitude seems to have remained
stable over time and to have existed before the diagnosis of MS. They
discussed their attitudes as though they were a permanent part of their
personality, for example:

My attitude, so many of my friends with MS have a very down attitude, a very miserable attitude . . . They have a debilitating disease

so they are debilitated. Well, I'm not . . . I've been told that I'm so amazingly wide open with my attitude I mean life goes on . . . (Pam)

> People call me the ultimate optimist. I think everything's going to be okay and I'm a great believer. If you really, really believe that way, you'll make it that way. (Barb)

On the other hand, Helen, a 67-year-old retired account representative, wife, and mother, feels that her life has become useless and out of her control:

> . . . Now I'll be quite truthful. I hope I don't live very long . . . I see the other people in our family who have been very active and they've been able to do things and participate and you know that type of thing. You know a useful life. And I don't see that for me.

Likewise, Xena, a 57-year-old retired dance instructor and single mother of four grown children, explains how MS has taken away her choices in life:

> Ever since I got the MS, it seems my life has just been giving me things to do . . . No choices. Survive the MS. Find a good doctor. How are you going to handle the MS? . . . It's like this is the time when the balls are being thrown at me. I'm not out there throwing the balls anymore.

Many participants described having a positive outlook on life as their most important coping strategy. Having an optimistic attitude about themselves and the world helped them focus on the good in their lives and deterred them from dwelling on negative elements. Others discussed viewing the world as a harsh environment in which they had no control. Those participants who seemed to have a negative outlook on life verbalized more feelings of helplessness and anger.

Another component of attitudinal perspectives that arose through the stories of the participants was the importance of faith and spirituality. Participants presented faith and spirituality as both an attitudinal perspective as well as a resource for specific action strategies that they used to cope with having multiple sclerosis. For example, faith and spirituality as an attitudinal perspective was discussed in terms of an emotional connection to a higher being that guides values and beliefs. In comparison, employing physical and emotional support received from one's religious community was discussed in terms of specific actions the participants took to cope. Carol's story illustrates both of these aspects of faith and spirituality.

Carol has a profound belief in God and is very involved with her Church. She spends much of her spare time (when she is feeling well) volunteering for Church sponsored charity events. Her congregation is her second family. As well as contributing to her positive attitude, Carol's faith helps her deal with the uncertainty of the future as a person aging with MS. Carol describes visiting a friend with MS who was living in a nursing home. Her friend had been diagnosed with MS at the same time Carol was, but her friend's disease had progressed much faster than Carol's. Carol reflects:

> I have a very strong faith, thank God. That did not leave me in the midst of all this other trauma. You know God can see them [people in the nursing home] as they truly are, as He created them to be. This is a temporary time and it's hard for them and when they're finished, when they die, they are going to be fully whole with Him. And if this happens to me, I can deal with it. It will be difficult but I can deal with it.

In contrast, Yolanda a 60-year-old retired medical secretary and wife, talks about her struggle with faith as a person with MS:

> But you can see [why], you get so depressed when you're, you know, and you can't walk anymore and do things. It's not fair. I think why does God do this to me? I say my prayers and I try so hard and this is what happens to me. It's not fair.

For some, strong faith in God seems to facilitate positive attitudes, and hope for the future. The belief that everything happens for a purpose and only God knows what that purpose is seems comforting to those who believe. For others, keeping faith in the face of aging with an unpredictable and chronic disease is a struggle. Through the process of practicing faith and spirituality, participants were also able to develop social networks. These networks will be discussed in more detail in the action strategies section.

Action Strategies

Action strategies are tasks that are physically carried out, actions taken that relieve stress. Three components of action strategies that were identified in the transcripts included: Seeking and using social supports; adapting environment; and planning for the future. Many of the action strategies that participants used reflected their attitudinal perspectives. Subsequently, there is some overlap in these two major themes and some examples presented below could be applied to both themes.

Like many of the participants interviewed for this study, Carol talked at great length about the important role her family and friends have played in supporting her throughout her life. Carol has an excellent social support network that contributes greatly to her positive attitude and feelings of self-efficacy. She is very close to her children and explains that she could not have gotten through the "tough times" without them.

As an example, Carol explained how her daughter purchased a house, keeping in mind that Carol may someday be unable to live on her own:

> When my daughter bought her house in [name of community], it has an extra bedroom on the main floor with a full bath and she said "now we got the house in particular in case you ever need to move in with us" which is the last thing in the world I want to do. But it's very reassuring to me just to know that that's there.

In contrast, Yolanda has been married for 26 years and does not have children. She describes her feelings about the lack of support she receives from her husband and how it affects their relationship:

> The main thing is when you have sickness, especially what I have, you have to get support from your husband. They don't understand. He says one day, last time I took care of you, you had diarrhea and stuff like that on purpose. He was so mad. You know what I mean? You have to be more understanding. I don't want to be like this. Do I want to lay here and have somebody wash me and take care of me? No. I want to take care of myself and do my own thing. I don't want it this way.

In addition to social support from her family, Carol is heavily involved with several MS support groups. Through them she has made many friends and feels she draws strength from her fellow members:

> I mean you're just yourself. And the same is true in the support group. People come as themselves. They're not afraid to share their weaknesses. They're proud of their strengths and they're so supportive of each other. It's made me less tolerant I think of phony people. But I don't know too many phony people.

Many other participants in the study expressed similar positive feelings about their experiences with support groups. For example, Elaine explains:

> We seem to understand each other's problems. So it does help us . . . You know, when you're around people who don't have MS, they really don't understand what MS is like. Just little things. So when you're around your own people that have the disease, you can talk freely and they can understand because they've been there.

Support groups helped participants cope in different ways. Whether it was giving, receiving or a combination of both, almost every person interviewed commented on the unique connection they developed with others who have MS. There seems to be a level of understanding and empathy present between those with the disease that is not possible in relationships with friends and family who do not have MS.

Another action strategy Carol uses that has helped her achieve independence and a positive outlook is adapting her physical environment to her needs. Her previous house had stairs that she had trouble climbing, and both full bathrooms were located on the second floor. Carol's present house is a one-level with wide hallways, open rooms, and a small yard. She bought the house, keeping in mind that she may need mobility aids at some point. She describes her thoughts about her present house:

> This is a nice house, and I like it too because I can live all on one floor. You know, when the MS hits, I could do it in this house. In fact, I noticed that most of the doorways are extra wide . . . So even if I had to have some kind of facility, a walker or even a wheelchair, I think that I would still be able to get around in here.

Other participants discussed the importance of modifying their existing homes, or planning moves to more accessible residences. Overall, participants were working to find or create accessible living spaces as they became more mobility challenged. Taking this action contributed to their self-sufficient and positive attitudes about where they live and what they are able to accomplish in their homes.

Another action strategy that Carol and other participants used to cope with MS was to look toward the future to predict and plan for their needs. For all of the participants, the anticipation of becoming severely disabled and losing independence helped frame the way they planned for the years ahead. Fears of not having enough money, becoming a burden, and living in a nursing home influenced their processes of planning for the future. Uncertain about how long she will be physically able to work, Carol has taken steps to plan for her financial future. She recently took a "planning for your retirement" course that has helped her make some important monetary decisions. Other participants talked about traveling now, before they became so disabled that travel would be too difficult or impossible to pursue.

In many of the plans that Carol and other participants discussed, the focus was on minimizing the burden their future care might place on family members. Becoming a burden was a major concern among participants, and coping with this concern directed many current strategies and future plans. For example, Beth, a 56-year-old married mother of five grown children, experienced a major exacerbation one year before the interview that left her severely disabled and very dependent on the help of her family. In response, Beth has hired a home health aide to help her as she becomes more disabled. She sees this assistance as managing her current needs, and also addressing the continued deterioration in her abilities in the future. At the time of the interview, her aide was working only on weekdays, and during other times her husband was providing for her care-taking needs. Beth talked about her fears of not being able to continue to afford the services of the aide:

> I have to pay for her . . . out of my own pocket, which is bad . . . it is finally getting to a point where [the money] is running out. My husband should be able to retire in four years. But we figure by that four years, I won't have enough money to pay for [my home health aide]. I'll be completely with no money.

For numerous participants, the fear of having to live in a nursing home helped steer their plans for the future. In many cases, they talked about nursing homes as the last choice, and some stated they would rather be dead:

> Yolanda: I want to stay in the house here as long as I can. I don't want to go to a nursing home. I've been in nursing homes and it's like a concentration camp and they tell you when to get up and when to go to bed . . . I want to stay here. I don't want to go to a nursing home.

The anticipation and fear of becoming more disabled and losing independence were important components in shaping participants' plans for the future.

DISCUSSION

The purpose of this study was to understand and describe coping processes used by women growing older with MS, from their own perspectives. While the original study from which the data used in this analysis included both men and women, only women were used in this analysis. Using the stories of the women, a model was created to make sense of the themes that emerged through the analysis of the qualitative interviews. Two major themes were found: Attitudinal perspectives and action strategies. Attitudinal perspectives incorporated four types of coping strategies: Sense of self, which included confidence in abilities and integration of MS; outlook on life; and practicing faith and spirituality. Action strategies contained three types of coping strategies: Seeking and using social supports; adapting environment; and planning for the future.

Overall examination of the transcripts suggested that those participants with positive attitudinal perspectives (e.g., had confidence in their abilities, integrated and accepted MS as a part of their lives, and had a positive outlook on life) seemed to employ more action strategies. This interpretation is in line with gerontological coping literature that reports successful adaptation to increases in physical limitation to be associated with positive and optimistic moods (Rubel, Reinsch, Tobis & Hurrell, 1994).

Coping literature also reports coping and perception of coping to be critical factors in dealing with chronic illness (Sinnakaruppan, 2000). However, the women in the current study discussed using denial as a coping strategy, and it appeared to be successful during long periods of remission as it limited excessive worry and stress about the disease. On the surface, this finding appears to contradict literature in which denial strategies are connected with increased risk of depression (Folkman et al., 1993; Lazarus, 1993). The difference may be in the use of language. For example, the women talked about being able to forget they had MS during periods of remission, which is more consistent with the notion of suppression (avoiding the problem) that is presented in the literature. Suppression has been found to be a positive coping strategy for people with chronic illness. While the women specifically used the term "denial" in their stories, it appears that the information that they were conveying is more consistent with the concept of suppression. Regardless of the label that is placed on this idea, the findings are consistent with studies that report avoidance and denial as positive coping strategies if they prevent the overwhelming stress of illness and disability (Shontz, 1975).

In the context of planning for the future as a coping strategy, participants discussed three main concerns they had about aging. These concerns stemmed from the anticipation of becoming severely disabled and losing independence. The major fears of not having enough money (inability to work), becoming a burden, and living in a nursing home all influenced participants' processes of planning for the future. The unpredictability of MS contributed to the urgency participants felt about making future plans. Gerontological literature reveals many of the same concerns among those aging in the general population, including fears of helplessness and being unable to manage one's life situation; illness and loss of independence; and physical disability (Nilsson, Sarvimäki & Ekman, 2000; Walker, 2000). In a study by the Alliance for Aging Research (1991), seventy-eight percent of adult respondents from a sample of 998 report they would prefer to die from sudden illness rather than live in a nursing home for many years.

This study can contribute to existing research in several ways. It brings to light the coping strategies, concerns and fears of people who are going through the experience of aging with MS. Studying those people who have had this chronic illness for many years uncovers distinct problems and suggests coping tools that arise from managing unpredictable disease symptoms and aging concurrently. Potentially, these findings can be used to develop and test interventions to teach people new coping strategies that include some of the strategies presented by the women interviewed. In addition, future researchers may want to examine changes in coping strategies over time in this population as it is unclear how the women developed the strategies that they discussed.

The findings of this research can inform practice by enabling occupational therapists as well as other healthcare practitioners to be more aware of the successful and unsuccessful coping strategies of this population, which can then be incorporated into treatment. Helping clients examine current coping skills, and initiating discussion of potential strategies can be a valuable tool in empowering people with MS to better manage their disease as they age. These discussions may help clients deal with mental health issues such as depression and anxiety. The use of coping strategies effects psychological symptoms (Aldwin &

Revenson, 1987). Therefore, identification of successful coping strategies is important because these tools have the potential to be taught and possibly halt or reverse the effects of depression and anxiety by improving confidence and self-efficacy. Introducing coping mechanisms that work may enable people to regain control and feel powerful in shaping the direction of their lives.

In addition, the qualitative nature of this study can contribute to a deeper understanding in health care professionals about what the experience of aging with MS is like. Qualitative research procedures are intended to unveil the meaning that the participants attach to phenomena, which may not be the same as definitions assigned by healthcare professionals (Marshall & Rossman, 1989; Strauss & Corbin, 1990).

Limitations of this study include the use of a small convenience sample, and the focus on women only. Participants were recruited through the Greater Illinois Chapter of the National Multiple Sclerosis Society. As a result, those aging with MS not associated with the Society were not given an equal opportunity to participate. Though the study was open to people of any ethnic or racial background who met the criteria, the sample was not diverse and consisted of all Caucasian participants. While the majority of people with MS are Caucasian (90%) (Minden, Marder, Harrold, & Dor, 1993), the experience of aging with the disease may not be the same for people of other racial or ethnic backgrounds. Gerontological research finds diverse populations to have unique concerns associated with growing older (Hunter, Linn, & Pratt, 1979). For these reasons, future research concerning those aging with MS who are from diverse racial and ethnic backgrounds is needed, and studies to explore differences between men and women would be valuable. Another limitation of this study is that the data were extracted from a larger study regarding service issues and health concerns among people aging with MS. Subsequently, there was not a specific agenda to look at coping strategies. The qualitative data could have been richer and more specific to coping if that had been the intent of the study.

CONCLUSION

This study intended to describe and provide a better understanding of the coping strategies of women aging with MS. The data support the conclusion that the women who integrate MS into their lives, have confidence in their abilities to cope with stress, and have a positive outlook on life, will use action strategies to cope with their disease. The overall findings suggest that attitude is linked with the types of coping strategies selected by the women aging with MS. This is important because simply teaching people new coping strategies may not be as successful when a discussion of attitude toward self and the world is ignored. The data also support the conclusion that women aging with MS have major concerns as they plan for their future and confront a range of fears including becoming more severely disabled and losing independence. The three most common fears discussed were financial stability, becoming a burden, and living in a nursing home. This study provides practitioners with a better awareness and understanding of the coping strategies, fears and concerns of those aging with MS. Further research is needed in order to clarify the uniqueness of coping strategies employed by those growing older with the disease, and to develop intervention strategies specific to this group's needs.

NOTE

1. The inventory includes the following instruments: Medical Outcomes Study Short Form (SF-36); Fatigue Impact Scale (FIS); MOS Pain Effects Scale (Derived from the Medical Outcomes Study Functioning and Well-Being Scale); Impact of Visual Impairment Scale; Self-Reported Cognitive Dysfunction: Perceived Deficits Questionnaire; Mental Health Inventory; and the Modified Medical Outcomes Social Support Survey.

REFERENCES

Aikens, J. E., Reinecke, M. A., Pliskin, N. H., Fischer, J. S., Wiebe, J. S., McCracken, L. M., & Taylor, J. L. (1999). Assessing depressive symptoms in multiple sclerosis: Is it necessary to omit items from the original Beck Depression Inventory? *Journal of Behavioral Medicine, 22*(2), 127-142.

Aldwin, C. M., & Revenson, T. A. (1987). Does coping help? A re-examination of the relation between coping and mental health. *Journal of Personality & Social Psychology, 53*(2), 337-348.

Alliance for Aging Research. (1991, November). *Americans View Aging: Results of a National Survey Conducted for the Alliance for Aging Research.* Washington, DC.

Bruce, M. L., Seeman, T. E., Merrill, S. S., & Blazer, D. G. (1994). The impact of depressive symptomatology on physical disability: MacArthur Studies of Successful Aging. *American Journal of Public Health, 84*(11), 1796-1799.

Christiansen, C.H., & Baum, C.M. (1997). *Occupational Therapy: Enabling Function and Well-being (2nd Edition).* Thorofare, NJ: Slack.

Downe-Wamboldt, B. L., & Melanson, P. M. (1998). A causal model of coping and well-being in elderly people with arthritis. *Journal of Advanced Nursing, 27*(6), 1109-1116.

Folkman, S., Chesney, M., Pollack, L., & Coates, T. (1993). Stress, control, coping, and depressive mood in human immunodeficiency virus positive and negative gay men in San Francisco. *Journal of Nervous and Mental Disease, 181(7),* 409-416.

Fournier, M., de Ridder, D., & Bensing, J. (1999). Optimism and adaptation to multiple sclerosis: What does optimism mean? *Journal of Behavioral Medicine, 22*(4), 303-326.

Hunter, K., Linn, M.W., & Pratt, T.C. (1979). Minority women's attitudes about aging. *Experimental Aging Research, 5*(2), 95-108.

Lazarus, R. S. (1993). Coping theory and research: Past, present, and future. *Psychosomatic Medicine, 55,* 234-247.

Malterud, K., Hollnagel, H., & Witt, K. (2001). Gendered health resources and coping: A study from general practice. *Scandinavian Journal of Public Health, 29*(3):183-188.

Marshall, C., & Rossman, G. (1989). *Designing Qualitative Research.* London: Sage.

Minden, S., Marder, W., Harrold, L., & Dor, A. (1993). *Multiple Sclerosis–A Statistical Portrait: A Compendium of Data on Demographics, Disability, and Health Services Utilization in the United States.* Cambridge, MA: Abt Associates.

Muhr, T. (1997) ATLAS.ti [Computer software]. Berlin: Scientific Software Development.

Nilsson, M., Sarvimäki, A., & Ekman, S. (2000). Feeling old: Being in a phase of transition in later life. *Nursing Inquiry, 7*(1), 41-49.

O'Neill, E. S., & Morrow, L. L. (2001). The symptom experience of women with chronic illness. *Journal of Advanced Nursing, 33*(2), 257-268.

Rubel, A. J., Reinsch, S., Tobis, J., & Hurrell, M. L. (1994). Adaptive behavior among elderly Americans. *Physical & Occupational Therapy in Geriatrics, 12*(4), 67-80.

Shontz, F. C. (1979). *The Psychological Aspects of Physical Illness and Disability.* New York: Macmillan.

Sinnakaruppan, I. (2000). Development of a coping scale for use with chronic illnesses, especially multiple sclerosis: A pilot study. *International Journal of Rehabilitation Research, 23(3),* 155-161.

Strauss, A., & Corbin, T. (1990). *Basics of Qualitative Research: Grounded Theory Techniques and Strategies.* Newbury Park, CA: Sage.

Sullivan, M. J., Mikail, S., & Weinshenker, B. (1997). Coping with a diagnosis of Multiple Sclerosis. *Canadian Journal of Behavioral Science, 29*(4), 249-257.

Walker, C. A. (2000). Aging among baby boomers. Unpublished doctoral dissertation, Texas Woman's University, Denton, Texas.

Wenger, G., Davies, R., & Shahtahmasebi, S. (1995). Morale in old age: Refining the model. *International Journal of Geriatric Psychiatry, 10*(11), 933-943.

Weinshenker, B. (1995). The natural history of multiple sclerosis. *Neurologic Clinics of North America, 13(1),* 119-146.

Occupational Therapy Practice and Research with Persons with MS: Final Reflections

Laura McKeown, BSc (Hons) OT, SROT (UK)
Marcia Finlayson, PhD, OT (C), OTR/L

Across the seven articles presented in this collection, authors have shared their work and offered suggestions about the potential implications for occupational therapy practice and research with persons with MS. We hope that you have found these articles to be stimulating and thought-provoking, and that the information gathered from them will be valuable to your work. We especially hope that you have enjoyed the international and multidisciplinary aspects of this volume.

As a wrap up to this special collection, we wanted to offer some of our own perspectives on the overarching themes we find across these seven articles, what these themes suggest about the current status of occupational therapy practice and research with persons with MS, and also what these themes suggest for future activities within our discipline.

Laura McKeown is a Postgraduate Research Student, Rehabilitation Sciences Research Group (Room 50K23), University of Ulster at Jordanstown, Newtownabbey, Co.Antrim, N. Ireland, BT37 OQB (E-mail: LP.McKeown@ulster.ac.uk).

Marcia Finlayson is Assistant Professor, Department of Occupational Therapy, University of Illinois at Chicago, 1919 W. Taylor Street, Chicago, IL 60612-7250 (E-mail: marciaf@uic.edu).

[Haworth co-indexing entry note]: "Occupational Therapy Practice and Research with Persons with MS: Final Reflections." McKeown, Laura, and Marcia Finlayson. Co-published simultaneously in *Occupational Therapy in Health Care* (The Haworth Press,) Vol. 17, No. 3/4, 2003, pp. 139-142; and: *Occupational Therapy Practice and Research with Persons with Multiple Sclerosis* (ed: Marcia Finlayson) The Haworth Press, Inc., 2003, pp. 139-142. Single or multiple copies of this article are available for a fee from The Haworth Document Delivery Service [1-800-HAWORTH, 9:00 a.m. - 5:00 p.m. (EST). E-mail address: docdelivery@haworthpress.com].

http://www.haworthpress.com/store/product.asp?sku=J003
10.1300/J003v17n03_09

The first theme that we see as emerging from these papers is the incredible complexity of MS as a disease, and the even more complex implications MS symptoms have for the people who live with them on a daily basis. We have read about the influence of tremor, using a wheelchair, fatigue and cognitive impairment. We have also read about how the complexity of MS does not decrease with age, but may even increase because of normal aging changes. The symptoms of MS are unpredictable and vary over time, cause a wide range of functional challenges, and often lead to the need for and use of a wide range of assistance, both paid (professional and paraprofessional) and unpaid (family and friends).

While most of the articles in the volume focus on professional assistance, many of them also highlight the need for occupational therapists to be attentive to family members, their support needs, and the importance of actively engaging them in any interventions that are being pursued with the person with MS. This is a second theme that we see as cutting across the articles in this volume. Although we do not have a paper that directly addresses family caregiving, the underlying thread in the articles presented is that occupational therapists who engage family members in the intervention process may enhance the likelihood of intervention success. However, a recent systematic literature review has demonstrated that few studies have been conducted specifically with caregivers with multiple sclerosis (McKeown, Porter-Armstrong & Baxter, 2003). Clearly this area requires more attention for both practitioners and researchers in our field.

A third theme that we saw across the articles included here is the need to expand our research efforts related to our work with persons with MS. Dr. LaRocca raises this point in his preface and then the theme continues throughout the volume. A number of the authors correctly describe their work as pilot or descriptive in nature, and point to the need to extend their efforts and use larger samples, more sophisticated measures, and more rigorous research designs. In addition, a number of the articles point to the importance of ensuring that both qualitative and quantitative perspectives are captured in MS-related inquiries. A recent editorial by Hasselkus (2003) states that qualitative research "seeks to understand the meaning of human phenomena, the nature of human experiences, and the dynamics of the processual elements of living" (p. 7). Indeed, the qualitative pieces included within this volume demonstrate that such research can provide occupational therapists with important insights into the lived experiences of persons with multiple sclerosis and their family members. The findings of qualitative research have great potential for broadening our perspectives on our interventions to ensure that they meet the needs of this diverse client group. Consistent with the recommendations of occupational therapy researchers (Kielhofner, Hammel, Finlayson, Helfrich, & Taylor, in press) and the recent report from the Institute of Medicine's Committee on Multiple Sclerosis (2001), many of the contributing authors call for researchers to develop and test, and for clinicians to employ, standardized assessment tools with sound psychometric properties. The benefits of this are two-fold. First, such tools will enable clinicians to reliably measure the effectiveness of their interventions, and second, if researchers employ the same assessment tools comparisons and pooling of data across studies will be possible. These strategies would strengthen our body of knowledge and provide empirical evidence about the best and most appropriate occupational therapy interventions for this client group.

It is important that readers remember that this special issue of represents a mere snapshot of the work that occupational therapists are currently pursuing within this field. A total of 17 manuscripts were reviewed and considered for this volume. Through the personal perspective of Dr. Gaetjens, and the articles included here, it is clear that occupational therapists can be instrumental in enabling persons with multiple sclerosis to manage their disease, work towards their occupational performance goals, and to engage in their communities to the highest extent possible. However, our profession is presented with the challenge to bridge "the gap" described by Dr. LaRocca. It is essential that we become active participants and contributors in the development and dissemination of knowledge related to MS not only within our own profession, but also with persons with multiple sclerosis, their families, and multidisciplinary clinicians and researchers. These efforts need to look to the future and the trends in occupational therapy and MS care. The directions for MS research outlined by the Institute of Medicine's Committee on Multiple Sclerosis (2001) are worth careful review as many of these recommendations fit with the ethos and goals of our profession.

In closing, we hope that this volume will become an important resource for occupational therapy students, clinicians and researchers who work with persons with multiple sclerosis and their families. It serves as an indicator of the current position of our profession in the MS field, and celebrates and highlights the importance of occupational therapy in enhancing the quality of life of individuals with this highly unpredictable chronic disease. This eclectic collection of articles points to an exciting future for both occupational therapy practice and research with persons with multiple sclerosis.

REFERENCES

Hasselkus, B.R. (2003). The voices of qualitative researchers: Sharing the conversation. *American Journal of Occupational Therapy, 57* (1), 7-8.

Institute of Medicine. (2001) *Multiple Sclerosis: Current Status and Strategies for the Future*. Washington, DC: National Academic Press.

Kielhofner, G., Hammel, J., Finlayson, M., Helfrich, C., & Taylor, R. (in press). Documenting outcomes of occupational therapy. *American Journal of Occupational Therapy*.

McKeown, L.P., Porter-Armstrong, A.P., & Baxter, G.D. (2003). The needs and experiences of caregivers of individuals with multiple sclerosis: A systematic review. *Clinical Rehabilitation, 17*, 234-248.

Index

Activities of daily living (ADLs),
    upper limb tremors in MS
    persons effects on, 81-95. *See
    also* Multiple sclerosis (MS),
    upper limb tremor in, effect
    on ADLs
Adaptability subscale score, 74
ADLs. *See* Activities of daily living
    (ADLs)
Aging
    as factor in MS, 116-117
    of women with MS, coping
        processes among, 115-137.
        See also Multiple sclerosis
        (MS), women aging with,
        coping processes among
ALS. *See* Amyotrophic lateral
    sclerosis (ALS)
Alusi, S.H., 83,91
Alzheimer's disease, 105
Amyotrophic lateral sclerosis (ALS),
    66
Armutlu, K., 92
Assistive devices, defined, 64
Assistive technology, defined, 64

Background Form for Wheelchairs, 68,
    69-70,70t-72t
Baker, N.A., 31
Barling, J., 97
Baum, C., 65
Baumhackl, U., 77
Beatty, W.W., 103
Bell, A., 3
Bennett, F., 40
Black, D.A., 22-23
Blake, R.L., 8

Bradshaw, J.L., 7
Brink, N., 106
Buchanan, D.C., 105

Canadian Occupational Performance
    Measure (COPM), 76
Chatto, C., 27
Chau, B., 63
CINAHL, 1
Clemmons, D.C., 40
Client factors
    defined, 29
    MS effects on, 29
Cognition, MS effects on, 102-103
College of Family Physicians of
    Canada, 32
Competency and Adaptation subscales,
    73
Consortium of Multiple Sclerosis
    Centers, 2
Coping
    among women aging with MS,
        115-137. *See also* Multiple
        sclerosis (MS), women aging
        with, coping processes
        among
    defined, 117
COPM. *See* Canadian Occupational
    Performance Measure
    (COPM)
Copperman, L.F., 40

DalMonte, J., 8,31,40,115
Davies, R., 118
Day, H., 66,68,73
Dehoux, E., 105

Demeres, L., 66,73,74
Dephoff, M., 97
Descent, M., 66
Devitt, R., 63
D'Hooghe, M., 45
Dickerson, A., 3
Downe-Wamboldt, B.L., 118
Drug(s), for MS, 116
Duportail, M., 45
Dyck, I., 40

EDSS. *See* Expanded Disability Status
       Scale (EDSS)
Eher, H., 77
European TREMOR Project, 91
European TREMOR Project DE3216,
       83
Expanded Disability Status Scale
       (EDSS), 84

FACES checklist, 58,59
FAI. *See* 29-item Fatigue Assessment
       Instrument (FAI)
FAMS. *See* Functional Assessment of
       Multiple Sclerosis (FAMS)
Fatigue
    defined, 102
    MS and, 102
       self-report assessment of. *See
       also* Multiple sclerosis (MS),
       fatigue in, self-report
       assessment of
Fatigue, MS and, 45-62
Fatigue Descriptive Scale (FDS), 49,
       51t,52t,55t
Fatigue Severity Scale (FSS), 49,51t,
       52t,55t
FDS. *See* Fatigue Descriptive Scale (FDS)
Feys, P., 81
FIM. *See* Functional Independence
       Measure (FIM)
Finlayson, M., 1,5,8,31,40,115,139
FIS. *See* 40-item Fatigue Impact Scale
       (FIS)

Fisher LSD procedures, 35
Flachenecker, P., 56
Fleming, S.T., 8
Ford, H.L., 65
40-item Fatigue Impact Scale (FIS),
       49,51t,52t,55t
Forwell, S.J., 40
Fournier, M., 118
Fraser, R.T., 40
Freeman, J.A., 8, 20, 22-23
Fruehwald, S., 77
FS. *See* Functional Systems (FS)
FSS. *See* Fatigue Severity Scale (FSS)
Functional Assessment of Multiple
       Sclerosis (FAMS), 50, 51t,
       52t,55t,57
Functional Independence Measure
       (FIM), 83,84,90
Functional Systems (FS), 86,87t,90

GASs. *See* Goal attainment scales
       (GASs)
Gerry, E., 65
Gillen, G., 30, 92
GNDS. *See* Guy's Neurological
       Disability Scale (GNDS)
Goal attainment scales (GASs), 111
Gryfe, P., 74
Guy's Neurological Disability Scale
       (GNDS), 50,51t,52t,55t,56-57

Harrisson, J., 83
Hasselkus, B.R., 140
Helfrich, H., 115
Hughes, M.L., 27
Hugos, L., 40
Human Assurance Committee, 32-33

IIRS. *See* Illness Intrusiveness Ratings
       Scale (IIRS)
Illness Intrusiveness Ratings Scale
       (IIRS), 50,51t,52t,55t,57

Institute of Medicine's Committee on Multiple Sclerosis, 141
Instrumentation, in study of coping processes among women aging with MS, 121
Intention tremor, defined, 82

Johnson, M.H., 65
Johnson, T., 97
Jones, L., 83, 92
Jongbloed, L., 40
Jutai, J., 63,66,73,74

Kerckhofs, E., 45
Kersten, P., 21
Ketelaer, P., 45,81
Kos, D., 45
Kraft, G.H., 23

Lapierre, Y., 73,74
LaRocca, 140,141
Lee, G.P., 27
Lewis, Y., 83
Lifestyle Management Programs (LMPs)
   described, 98-99
   in persons with MS, 97-114
      case example, 107-110,109f, 110f
      development of, 101-104
      implementation of, 101-104
      literature review related to, 104-106
      study of
         background of, 99-100
         introduction to, 98-100
LMPs. *See* Lifestyle Management Programs (LMPs)
Loeffler-Stastka, H., 77

"Managing Fatigue," 106

Mann-Whitney U test, 33
Masku Neurological Rehabilitation Centre, 84, 85
Mateer, C.A., 105
Mathiowetz, V., 30,106
Matsumoto, J., 83
Matuska, K.M., 106
McKeown, L., 139
MEDLINE, 1
Melanson, P.M., 118
MFIS. *See* Modified Fatigue Impact Scale (MFIS)
Mini Mental Scale, 85-86
Mini Mental State Examination (MMSE), 84
MMSE. *See* Mini Mental State Examination (MMSE)
Modified Fatigue Impact Scale (MFIS), 49,51t,52t,55t,102
Monette, M., 66,73,74
Mosley, L.J., 27
Movement Disorders Society, 82
MS. *See* Multiple sclerosis (MS)
MS Council for Clinical Practice Guidelines (MSCCPG), 105-106
MS Society of NSW, 101
MSCCPG. *See* MS Council for Clinical Practice Guidelines (MSCCPG)
MSS-FS. *See* Multiple Sclerosis Specific-Fatigue Scale (MSS-FS)
Multiple sclerosis (MS)
   aging effects on, 116-117
   client factors influenced by, 29-30
      interventions for, 30-31
   clinical signs in, 29-30
   cognitive changes in, 102-103
   defined, 6,28,64
   described, 82,116
   drugs for, 116
   fatigue in, 102
      evaluation of, 47,48t
      prevalence of, 46

self-report assessment of, 45-62
    discussion of, 57-58
    implications for, 57-58
    instrumentation in, 49-50,51t
        evaluation of, 50-57,51t,
            52t,55t
    introduction to, 46-47,48t
    method of, 49
    results of, 49-57,51t,52t,55t
LMPs in, 97-114. *See also* Lifestyle
    Management Programs
    (LMPs), in persons with MS
occupational therapy for, 27-43
    implications for, 40-41
    practice of, 139-142
    research related to, 139-142
    study of
        data analysis in, 33
        discussion of, 38-41
        functional implications of,
            36-38, 39t
        introduction to, 28-32
        limitations of, 41
        participants in, 32, 33-34,35t
        purpose of, 28-29
        results of, 33-38,35t-37t,39t
        survey instrument in, 32-33
        symptom analysis in, 34-36,
            35t,36t
older adults with
    health service need, use, and
            variability of, study
            of, 5-25
        analysis of, 13
        design of, 9-13, 12t
        discussion of, 19-23
        factors influencing utilization
            of, 17-19,18t
        instrumentation in, 11-13,12t
        introduction to, 6
        literature review related to, 7-9
        methods in, 9-13,12t
        participants in, 10-11
        procedures of, 11-13,12t
        results of, 13-19,14t,16t, 18t

health-related service needs of,
    15-17,16t
    interpretation of, 13,14t
    image of, 14-15
progression of, 28
symptoms of, 116
upper limb tremor in, effect on
        ADLs, 81-95
    study of
        data analysis in, 85
        data collection in, 84-85
        discussion of, 90-92
        findings from standard scales
            in, 86,87t,88t
        methods in, 83-85
        participant(s) in, 83-84,85-86
        participant survey findings in,
            86,88-90,89t
        procedures in, 84-85
        results of, 85-90,87t-89t
        standard scales in, 84
        survey in, 84-85
wheelchair use for persons with,
    quality of life effects of, 63-79
    study of
        analysis of, 69
        discussion of, 73-77
        introduction to, 64-67
        method in, 67-69
        outcome measure in,
            67-68
        participants in, 67
        procedure for, 68-69
        results of, 69-73,70t,
            71f, 71t, 72f
women aging with, coping
        processes among, 115-137
    literature review related to,
            117-118
    study of
        action strategies in,
            129-133
        analysis of, 121-122
        attitudinal perspectives in,
            125-129

case example, 122, 124-133
design of, 119-122,120t
discussion of, 133-135
instrumentation in, 121
methods in, 119-122,120t
participants in, 119,120t
procedures in, 119,121
results of, 122-133,123f
Multiple Sclerosis Council for Clinical
Practice Guidelines
(MSCCPG), 102
Multiple Sclerosis Quality of Life
Inventory, 49,51t,52t,55t,121
Multiple Sclerosis Society of New
South Wales, Australia, 97,98
Multiple Sclerosis Specific-Fatigue
Scale (MSS-FS), 49-50,51t,
52t,55t
Multiscale Depression Inventory, 57
Murphy, M.E., 106

Nagels, M., 45
National Centre for Multiple Sclerosis,
Melsbroek, 83-84, 85
National Multiple Sclerosis Society
(NMSS), 1,10,21,118,119
Greater Illinois Chapter of, 135
1964 Declaration of Helsinki, 85
NMSS. *See* National Multiple
Sclerosis Society (NMSS)
Northwick Park ADL Index, 83
Nuyens, G., 45
Nygard, L., 105

OARS. *See* Older Americans
Resources and Services
Questionnaire (OARS)
Occupational Performance Model
(Australia) [OPM (A)], 99
Occupational therapy, for MS, 27-43.
See also Multiple sclerosis
(MS), occupational therapy for

*Occupational Therapy Practice
Framework: Domain and
Process,* 29
Ohman, A., 105
Older Americans Resources and
Services Questionnaire
(OARS), 121
OPM (A). *See* Occupational
Performance Model
(Australia) [OPM (A)]
OTDBASE, 1

Packer, T.L., 106
Paulsson, E.H., 32
PEO Model. *See* Person-Environment-
Occupation (PEO) Model
Person-Environment-Occupation
(PEO) Model, 76
PIADS. *See* Psychosocial Impact of
Assistive Devices Scale
(PIADS)
Psychosocial Impact of Assistive
Devices Scale (PIADS),
63-64,66,67,68,70,71f,72f
Caregiver (proxy) Version of, 75
clinical utility of, 74-75
incorporation into occupational
therapy practice, 75-77
limitations of, 76-77
results with, 70-73,71f,72f

Quality of life, wheelchair use among
MS patients effects on,
63-79. *See also* Multiple
sclerosis (MS), wheelchair
use for persons with, quality
of life effects of

Rand Index of Vitality (RIV), 56
Rand's Health Insurance Survey, 56
RIV. *See* Rand Index of Vitality (RIV)
Roessler, C., 97

Romberg, A., 81
Ruutiainen, J., 81

Saletu, B., 77
Sauriol, A., 106
Schwid, S.R., 54
Screening Examination for Cognitive
    Impairment, 103
SF-36. *See* Short Form-36 (SF-36)
Shahtahmasebi, S., 118
Shevil, E., 5
Shontz, F.C., 117
Short Form-36 (SF-36),50,51t,52t,55t
Sinnakaruppan, I., 117
Soderback, I., 32
Sohlberg, M.M., 105
Somerset, M., 21
Stolp-Smith, K., 8
Study Advisory Group member, 10
Sullivan, M.J.L., 105,117
Sweeney, S., 97

Tennant, A., 65
Thompson, A.J., 8,20,22-23,31
Tickle-Degenen, L., 31
Tremor(s)
    intention, defined, 82
    upper limb, MS-related, effect on
        ADLs, 81-95. *See also*

Multiple sclerosis (MS),
    upper limb tremor in, effect
    on ADLs
29-item Fatigue Assessment
    Instrument (FAI), 49-50,51t,
    52t,55t

Upper limb, tremors of, MS-related,
    effect on ADLs, 81-95. *See*
    also Multiple sclerosis (MS),
    upper limb tremor in, effect
    on ADLs

Van Denend, T., 5
VAS. *See* Visual analogue scale (VAS)
Visual analogue scale (VAS), 56

Wenger, G., 118
Wheelchair(s), for persons with MS,
    quality of life effects of,
    63-79. *See also* Multiple
    sclerosis (MS), wheelchair
    use for persons with, quality
    of life effects of
Wiles, C.M., 83
Wolfson, C., 66
World Federation of Occupational
    Therapists, 2